# DIET 2000

Dr Alan Maryon-Davis qualified at St Thomas's Hospital,
London, and spent several years as a hospital doctor before
specialising in preventive medicine. He joined the Health
Education Council in 1977 and was closely involved with its
'Look After Yourself!' Campaign – the first major campaign to
improve the British diet. He is currently Chief Medical Officer
with the Council and coordinator of its heart disease prevention
programme.

Dr Maryon-Davis is a frequent broadcaster and writer on health
matters and became familiar to many as the resident doctor on
BBC Radio One's 'Staying Alive' programmes. He also
presented the BBC Radio 4 series 'Action Makes the Heart Grow
Stronger'. In his spare time he enjoys eating good food and
singing with the humorous group 'Instant Sunshine'. He lives
with his wife and daughter in Clapham.

Jane Thomas obtained a BSc in Nutrition at London University
in 1971 and went on to Montreal, where she obtained her
postgraduate qualification in dietetics. Following completion of
a Master of Medical Science degree, she joined the Health
Education Council in 1974 and was their Research Officer until
1979 when she took up the post of Lecturer in Social Nutrition
at Queen Elizabeth College, University of London. In addition
to writing and broadcasting on the subject of healthy eating, her
other activities include bringing up her two young children in
Oxford where she lives with her dentist husband.

# DIET 2000

## At last – a diet you can live with

Dr Alan Maryon-Davis
with Jane Thomas

**Pan Original**
Pan Books London and Sydney

First published 1984 by Pan Books Ltd,
Cavaye Place, London SW10 9PG
9 8 7 6 5 4 3 2 1
© Dr Alan Maryon-Davis 1984
ISBN 0 330 28628 5
Photoset by Parker Typesetting Service, Leicester
Printed and bound in Great Britain by
Richard Clay (The Chaucer Press) Ltd, Bungay, Suffolk

# Contents

# Acknowledgements

We would like to express our thanks to Professor Philip James of the Rowett Research Institute, Aberdeen, and principal author of the NACNE Report, for inspiring us to translate the Report into popular everyday language.

We would also like to thank the following for their helpful advice: Professor Jerry Morris, Emeritus Professor of Community Health, London University, and Chairman of the National Advisory Committee on Nutrition Education (NACNE); Dr David Player, Director-General of the Health Education Council; Dr John Brown, Research and Development Officer, Health Education Council; Dr Pat Judd, Nutritionist, Queen Elizabeth College, London; Derek Miller, Nutritionist, Queen Elizabeth College, London; Caroline Walker, Nutritionist, St Bartholomew's Hospital, London.

Very special thanks go to Hilary Davies of Pan for liking the original idea and bringing it so enthusiastically to fruition, and to Annie Jackson, also of Pan, who skilfully knocked it all into shape.

Finally, much love and gratitude to our respective spouses for each holding the fort so stoically whilst the typewriters clattered away.

The Diet 2000 Food Score Table is based largely on the analyses published in McCance and Widdowson's *The Composition of Foods* (4th edn) by A. A. Paul and D. A. T. Southgate, HM Stationery Office, London.

The charts on the current British diet are based on data from the National Food Survey conducted by the Ministry of Agriculture, Fisheries and Food.

The NACNE Report is published by the Health Education Council.

While the dietary principles and targets used in this book are based on the NACNE Report, the views we express are entirely our own.

# Introduction:
# the great breakthrough

## Yet another diet book?

No, this is *not* just another of those diet books that cram the shelves of your local bookshop. This is *not* the latest in a long line of 'miracle breakthrough' diets for slimmers. This is *not* another bid to join the ranks of the Scarsdale diet, the Pritikin diet, the Beverley Hills diet, or the F-Plan diet. In fact this isn't a diet book at all if you think of diets only in terms of 'dieting' – losing as much flab as you can.

This book is about something much more crucial than your waistline or winning the battle with the bathroom scales – important though that certainly is for some people. So many people are so concerned with their looks and their figures that they forget or deliberately choose to ignore something they probably take for granted. Something which is more important to happiness than almost everything else.

Good health.

When you weigh it all up, the average person in the well-fed nations of the West eats about half a ton of food a year. And then there's all the drink on top of that. So it's hardly surprising that what you eat can have a profound effect, not just on your weight, but on your health. And that means not only your health right now, but also your health – and your family's health – in years to come.

So, this book is about healthy eating for you and your family.

But much more than that. It's about a revolution in nutrition – a brand new set of dietary guidelines formulated by a panel of top scientific experts to get us eating more healthily by the year 2000. It is a blueprint for change. The diet of tomorrow for each and every one of us. Young or old, male or female, fat or thin – we can all benefit from the shift to a healthier way of eating.

But why wait till tomorrow?

The time to start on the right tracks is now.

This book gives you the facts behind the new diet. It explains in simple straightforward language how eating can affect your health, and the principles involved in changing for the better.

1

It sets out clear guidelines and targets to aim at. It gives you easy-to-follow charts and tables. And to dispel any doubts you may have about whether it'll ruin your appetite, there are recipes galore showing just how delicious healthy meals can be.

## So, what's new?

There have been books on healthy eating before. But until now they've all suffered from one major drawback. Although they may advise you to eat less of this or more of that, they've never actually told you *how much* less or *how much* more. True, the slimming books have usually set down some very specific rules in the form of a day-to-day or week-by-week dieting plan. But leaving slimming books aside, the books that have advised on eating for general good health have merely been saying 'cut down on fat' or 'eat more fruit and vegetables' without giving any real clue as to what they mean by 'cut down' or 'eat more'. One ounce of butter less each week, or four? An extra apple a day, or several? How much sugar? What about salt?

We believe this book breaks new ground because it sets you clear, precise targets based on the recently published report of a top-level panel of scientific experts. Using these guidelines you can at last plan your eating habits to get the mixture right on target as far as your health is concerned.

## Why have we had to wait so long?

This isn't just another fashion in eating, here one minute and gone the next, like grapefruit with everything, or thrice daily yogurt, or pineapple till it comes out of your ears, or bran till your jaws are aching. This is a nutritional guide based on painstaking scientific research, the end result of years of careful experiment and observation by teams of nutritional, biochemical, epidemiological and other experts from many parts of the world. Their work has been checked and sifted, analysed and ordered, and drawn together in a series of major reports on various aspects of food and health.

Just recently came the biggest step forward of all. A document so modest in its intentions that the experts who compiled it and presented it for publication merely hoped that it would stimulate discussion among the various professional groups who are concerned with nutrition education. It certainly achieved that. But it achieved rather more than that. In fact, its proposals were so far-reaching in nutritional planning that the so-called 'discussion paper' turned out to be nothing less than a bombshell. It has shaken the steady world of dietetics, home economics, food marketing, and agricultural planning to the very roots as more and more dieticians and nutritionists begin to put its proposals into practice. And now its principles are reaching the general public – reaching you – with this simple guide to the 'new' diet.

# The NACNE Report

The modest report that has set the nutritional world alight, and forms the basis for this book, has become known as 'The NACNE Report' (pronounced 'knack-knee') after the UK National Advisory Committee on Nutrition Education, the committee which commissioned it. In fact the report was the result of the work of a panel of doctors, nutritionists, and education experts under the chairmanship of Professor W. P. T. James, Director of the Rowett Research Institute, Aberdeen, and a leading nutritional scientist of international repute.

Even with this impressive array of expertise the NACNE Report does not claim to have come up with any startling new discovery, like some hitherto unknown food factor or vital vitamin or fundamental nutritional principle. Indeed the report's great strength is that it is firmly based on a number of other publications, all of them major official, academic or international reports of the highest standards of scientific objectivity. Just look at the list:

- The UK Department of Health's report 'Eating for Health'.
- The UK Department of Health's report 'Diet and Coronary Heart Disease'.
- The UK Department of Health's report 'Avoiding Heart Attacks'.
- The UK Department of Health's report 'Recommended daily amounts of food energy and nutrients for groups of people in the United Kingdom'.
- The Royal College of Physicians and British Cardiac Society report 'The Prevention of Coronary Artery Disease'.
- The Royal College of Physicians report 'Medical Aspects of Dietary Fibre'.
- The Royal College of Physicians report 'Obesity'.
- The World Health Organisation report 'The Prevention of Coronary Heart Disease'.

All these reports made recommendations on various aspects of nutrition and health. But NACNE goes one step further. It brings them all together as a set of proposals laying down clear guidelines as to just how, *and by how much*, we need to change our eating habits to enjoy healthier and longer lives.

## So why hasn't NACNE made the bestseller list?

The one unfortunate thing about the NACNE report is that it is written in technical language and aimed deliberately at professionals working in the field of nutrition education. As it stands it is quite useless to the layman. It needs to be translated into everyday terms that the public at large can understand. Which is why we've produced Diet 2000.

The book is in two parts.

The first is a simple summary of the main points from the NACNE report, covering such important aspects as:

- the 'balanced' diet;
- body weight and health;
- dietary fat and coronary heart disease;
- dietary fibre and bowel disorders;
- salt and blood pressure;
- sugar and dental health;

and giving the key NACNE guidelines in a form that makes sense to those without a degree in nutritional science, but who nevertheless are entrusted with the literally vital task of choosing, cooking and eating food.

The second part puts theory into practice by helping you apply the NACNE formula to your eating choice – in the shops, in the kitchen and at the table. With the help of its simple but comprehensive charts, you can choose what to buy, how to prepare and whether to eat the food that can so fundamentally affect your health. And with the help of its specially adapted recipes, you can cook a whole range of nutritious and appetizing meals.

# Part One:
# Why Diet 2000?

## What on earth is a 'balanced' diet?

No doubt you've heard the phrase 'balanced' diet often enough to drive you off balance trying to work out what it can possibly mean! We all know we should eat a balanced diet, but what is balanced with what? The meat with the mash? The peas with the pudding? The butter with the baked beans? Or is it all to do with getting enough protein? Or vitamins and minerals? Or energy?

The whole idea of the balanced diet began back in the days when the biggest nutritional problem facing us was that of going short of vital nutrients. The most important thing in those days was to make sure that everybody, particularly children, pregnant women and the elderly, got enough protein, vitamins and minerals to keep them healthy. And that meant that meals needed to be 'balanced' by using foods of different types that would provide varied sources of these vital nutrients. So 'balance' essentially meant variety. And 'variety' essentially meant getting enough of a mixture of different types of foods.

But nowadays hardly anyone in the West is in danger of going short of essential nutrients. We now have such a wide variety of foods available to us, reasonably cheaply, that it is only people on very inadequate diets – such as people on low incomes, some food faddists and elderly people living alone who can't do enough shopping or cooking – who are possibly missing out on certain vitamins.

No, getting enough isn't the problem these days. The average person's diet contains more than enough. On the contrary, today's big nutritional problem is that we're eating much too much of certain types of food. Our diet has become unbalanced in a rather different way from the unbalanced diet of the old days. It is now overloading us. And in doing so it is putting a strain on certain important body mechanisms.

- *Too many calories* means putting on weight, and that can increase the risk of getting high blood pressure, diabetes and heart disease.

- *Too much fat* (apart from the calories it contains) means unbalancing the fatty substances carried in the bloodstream. And that can lead to deposits of fatty material on the inner lining of the arteries, which can cause heart disease.
- *Too much sugar* (apart from the calories it contains) encourages bacteria in the mouth, altering the acidity and leading to tooth decay. Also high 'doses' of sugar may play a part in causing gallstones and diabetes.
- *Too much salt* can push up the blood pressure and hence increase the risk of getting heart disease or a stroke.

Nevertheless, there is one important food item that we are *not* getting enough of these days. Something that doctors and nutritionists have only recently started to appreciate as a very necessary part of a healthy diet. Something which used to be dismissed as mere padding or 'roughage', just passing through. That 'something' is of course what we now know as dietary fibre.

- *Too little dietary fibre* slows down the digestive processes and can cause bowel disorders. Without the low-calorie bulk of fibre in our food we tend to eat too much of the fatty and sugary foods. In other words our appetite-control mechanism becomes unbalanced and that, for many of us, means we gain weight.

While we're on the subject of the 'balanced' diet, the importance of variety and the need to eat less of some sorts of food and more of others, there is another important principle that we should mention. And that is – to take a broad view of what you're eating. What do we mean by that?

Too many people get so finnicky about the health aspects of individual items in their day-to-day food that they lose sight of what their diet *as a whole* is doing for their health. They can't see the wood for the trees. They think of this or that item as either a 'good' food or a 'bad' food and then proceed either to eat as much of it as they decently can or avoid it like the plague. This attitude is not only short-sighted, it's also wrong. To eat a chocolate éclair when you're overweight is not the end of the world. In fact it needn't make a jot of difference providing you cut down the rest of your eating by an equal number of calories. To tuck into a buttered bun or bacon and eggs is not another nail in your coffin due to heart disease, providing you cut down on saturated fats in your diet overall.

It's the *totality* of the diet that counts.

And it's the little excesses that make life worth living. Critics will say that if you give people an inch they will take a mile. But we believe that with enough information people can work out for themselves whether they should or shouldn't eat that particular chocolate éclair or this plate of bacon and eggs.

And we believe that Diet 2000 will give you the advice you need to make the right food choices for your long-term health.

Later in this book we'll be looking a little more closely at fat, fibre, sugar and salt, and their effects on health. But first let's consider calories, because as every slimmer knows only too well balancing your calorie intake with your energy output is the key to fighting the flab. And too much body fat isn't just a question of how you look, or how you feel, it's also an important factor in your health. Now and later on.

# Dying for a bite: how we are eating our way to ill health

## *Overweight: tipping the scales against your health*

The yearning for a slim, trim figure has become such a universal obsession that there is now a multi-million-pound industry catering for the avid slimmer's every need. Indeed, some would say that the preoccupation with being 'fat', and the guilt surrounding it, is bordering on mass hypochondria and causing a great deal of needless misery for millions. The worst thing about being overweight, they say, is worrying about it.

But quite apart from what that surplus stone or two might, or might not, be doing to one's looks or self-confidence, the sad fact is that *obesity can seriously damage your health*.

Now that probably comes as no surprise to you because it's long been known that being very fat ('obese' means being at least twenty per cent heavier than the top end of the 'desirable' weight range for the person's height) increases the risk of suffering a long list of ills, including coronary heart disease (heart attack or angina), hypertension (high blood pressure), diabetes, gallbladder disease, back trouble, arthritis, chest problems, varicose veins, and painful feet – to say nothing of the general discomfort and embarrassment caused by having to cart about a great bulk and weight.

But what perhaps is rather more surprising is that, according to the Royal College of Physicians' recent report on obesity, even being just a few pounds overweight can start to tip the scales against your future health, especially if you're under thirty, and even more especially if you're male.

The life insurance statistics of hundreds of thousands of American men and women have been analysed to see if there is a link between body weight and longevity. The answer is that for people who become overweight before the age of fifty and stay that way there is a definite extra risk of an early death. Just how great the risk is depends on how much overweight you are and how long you've been like that. The heavier you are, and the longer you've been straining the scales, the more likely you are to die young. Being a few pounds over the weight range 'desirable' for your height will only add a little extra risk – but extra risk it is nonetheless, especially if you're fairly young.

Now this all sounds rather alarming. Could your cuddly spare tyre really be a killer? Or your podgy thighs a potential hazard to life? Isn't this just yet more scaremongering by the medical fraternity?

The explanation is that mild degrees of overweight in youth all too often mean great rolls of the stuff later in life, with all its attendant disadvantages. What's more, for people with a family tendency to high blood pressure, diabetes or heart disease, a few extra pounds can make all the difference as to whether, when or how these problems develop.

## Everybody's different

Averages are all very well, but what makes life interesting is that everybody's different. We all inherit different body shapes, different metabolisms, different rates of ageing. And we have different lifestyles, with different eating and drinking habits, taking different amounts of exercise, coping with different degrees of stress, and indulging in different vices.

All these factors affect our nutritional balance and in particular our need for calories. It is one of life's fundamental injustices that some people can stuff themselves silly with all manner of fatty and sugary excesses without gaining an ounce, whilst others have only to peep at a profiterole and they put on pounds.

Over the past few years, scientists have begun to unravel the mystery of how our bodies differ so widely in the way they cope with extra calories.

One basic difference is our sex. Normal-weight women have about fifty per cent more body fat than normal-weight men. That's thanks to evolution. The extra fat not only gives women their characteristic curves but also provides them with a reserve energy supply that could, in times of famine, keep them alive and able to suckle their infants. Men are leaner and more muscular which, in evolutionary terms, made them better equipped for their role as hunter-gatherers and in fighting off enemies and predators.

And of course the other big difference is in the level of physical activity. The harder you work the more calories you burn up, in just the same way as a car that's driven faster burns more petrol. Also the bigger your muscles, the more calories they need to get them moving; so active men burn up more calories than equally active women. It isn't fair, is it?

Another way we all differ from each other is in the 'tickover' or 'idling speed' of our metabolism (called the 'basal metabolic rate') which determines how fast we burn up calories just doing nothing – in other words the calories required to fuel all our various body processes whilst we're at rest. There is some evidence that people who need fewer calories to tick over are more likely to get fat easily.

There seems to be a way in which some people can speed up their basal metabolic rate and that's by taking *regular* exercise. Scientists are discovering that regular exercisers – who exert themselves fairly vigorously for 20–30 minutes, two or three times a week – actually increase their body's tickover speed so that they burn up more calories even when they're resting. Unfortunately, it doesn't seem to work for everybody. But there are some lucky souls who, providing they make the necessary effort during the day, can actually slim while they sleep!

Another factor is the body's central heating system, called thermogenesis. This is a mechanism for dissipating excess calories in the form of heat. Lean people are better at it than fat people; and it could explain their difference in weight. If a naturally thin person is fed a high calorie meal, their body responds by generating more heat; rather as if they had switched from being a one-bar to a two-bar electric fire. But a person who is prone to overweight, even though he or she may be slim at the time, will respond to the meal by laying down fatty tissue.

All this goes to show that staying slim and losing excess weight is a very individual matter. If you have a weight problem it's very much a case of tailoring a diet to suit *you*.

This is why we think you'll find the advice in Diet 2000 so useful. Because it's *flexible* where it needs to be flexible – in letting you choose the energy intake that fits your circumstances. But *firm* where it needs to be firm – in making sure that not too many of your calories come from fatty or sugary foods.

## There's a lot of it about

According to the Royal College of Physicians, Britain is getting fatter. About one adult in three is overweight; rather more of them men than women. As you've probably discovered, body fat has a way of creeping up on you as you get older. Whilst about 15 per cent of teenagers are overweight, the proportion rises to over half of the nation's pensioners. This is not because getting fat is a normal part of the ageing process, but partly because your body chemistry changes as you get older and partly because you tend to be rather less physically active. Either way your body needs fewer calories but it's all too easy not to make the necessary changes to your diet.

The trend that really concerns the doctors is that more and more people in their twenties are overweight, and it's been suggested that this may be linked to the recent 'fast-food' boom, with so many young people living on burgers, fried chicken legs and chips with everything.

## Check your weight here

Obviously your weight depends mainly on your height (hence the familiar excuse 'I'm not fat . . . I'm just too short for my weight'). So here are height/weight charts based on the 'official' tables presented in the NACNE Report.

Weigh yourself without clothes and measure your height without shoes. To use the chart run one finger across from your height and another up from your weight. Where the fingers touch read off which weight category you are in.

*Underweight*  Are you eating enough?
*Desirable*  Stay right where you are
*Overweight*  Your health could suffer, start slimming down
*Obese*  It's very important for you to lose weight

**Men**

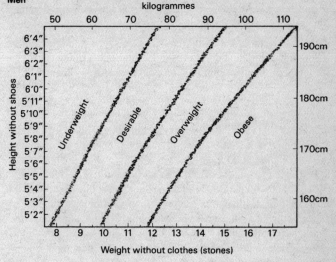

kilogrammes

Height without shoes

Underweight  Desirable  Overweight  Obese

Weight without clothes (stones)

**Women**

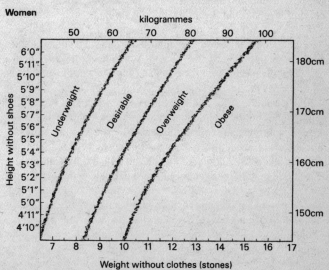

kilogrammes

Height without shoes

Underweight  Desirable  Overweight  Obese

Weight without clothes (stones)

13

## Fatty food and your heart

Coronary heart disease is the single biggest killer in the Western world. More than one person in four dies of coronary heart disease, usually in the form of a heart attack. It claims the lives of nearly half the men who die in middle age. And although it's less of a scourge for women, they've recently been going through a coronary 'epidemic' too.

Coronary heart disease doesn't always mean sudden death. All too often it leads to chronic ill health, either in the form of ever-worsening heart attacks or as the crippling chest pain called angina.

But however it strikes, heart disease is a dangerous, frightening *and largely preventable* condition.

Britain (or more particularly Scotland and Northern Ireland) is at the top of the international league table for heart disease deaths. Its heart disease death rate is over six times greater than the rate in Japan, which is at the bottom of the league. What's more, while the death rate in Britain is only just beginning to subside, there has already been a massive drop in heart disease deaths in several Western countries, including the US, Canada, Australia, New Zealand, Finland and Belgium.

Why should there be such big differences between countries? And why are some clearly winning the battle against heart disease whilst others, such as Britain, aren't? As you might imagine there's been a lot of research into the possible causes of heart disease in an effort to answer these questions.

All the experts agree that heart disease is not caused by any one single thing, but by a combination of different 'risk factors'. Some of the risk factors you can do nothing about – like your age (the older you are, the greater your risk of heart disease), your sex (men are between four and five times more likely to be killed by heart disease in middle age than are women) and your genes (you might inherit a resistance, or a susceptibility, to heart disease). But other risk factors are linked to your everyday habits – like whether you eat a fatty diet (too much fat, particularly saturated fat, puts up the risk), smoke (the average cigarette smoker has double the risk of a heart attack), or don't take enough regular exercise (20–30 minutes a time, two or three times a week, moderately vigorous exercise can halve the risk of a heart attack).

## Fat: sowing the seeds of heart disease

The fundamental flaw that leads to heart disease is the gradual 'furring up' of the narrow coronary arteries, which supply blood to the heart itself, with a fatty deposit called atheroma. This process usually takes decades before the coronaries are so clogged that they cause a heart attack or angina. But the disturbing fact is that *it often begins in childhood*. Young teenagers killed in accidents have been found to have streaks of fatty atheroma in their arteries. It is a grave mistake to think of heart disease as 'a bolt from the blue' that strikes people down in later life – or doesn't, depending on 'the luck of the draw'. The seeds of heart disease are sown at a very early age. Much earlier than most people realise – including parents. If only more parents were aware of the risks of feeding their children with a very fatty diet, there would be many fewer victims of heart disease beyond the year 2000.

## Saturated? polyunsaturated? . . . gobbledygook?

Worldwide studies have shown a striking link between heart disease statistics and the amount of fat in the diet. And the strongest link seems to be with a particular kind of fat, the real villain in the heart disease story, *saturated fat*.

According to various studies of different populations throughout the world, the proportion of saturated fat in the diet is closely linked to the death rate for heart disease. So the overall conclusion is that *a diet high in saturated fat is more likely to cause heart disease than a diet low in saturated fat*. Controlled dietary experiments have shown that a high saturated fat diet tends to push up the level of fatty substances in the blood (blood cholesterol), more in some people than in others, depending on their genes. And people with a high blood cholesterol level are more likely to have a heart attack or angina, again depending on their genes.

The fat in your food is not just one single chemical substance. There are many different sorts of fat. For instance, some fats are quite solid or hard at room temperature – such as lard, butter and hard margarines. Others are liquid and are called oils – such as corn oil, olive oil and sunflower oil. A third category are a blend of hard and liquid fats which appear as a soft 'grease' – such as soft margarines. All these fats are equally fattening because they all have the same number of calories. But because they have different chemical structures, they have different effects on your body.

In fact the chemistry is very complicated and we needn't here go into precisely what the biochemists mean by the terms 'saturated' and 'polyunsaturated'. All you really need to know is that some kinds of fat are more 'saturated' than others. These more saturated fats are found mostly in meat and dairy products and also most margarines. The less saturated fats (sometimes referred to as 'unsaturated' fats) are found mostly in vegetable oils. So broadly speaking, saturated fats are mostly of animal origin while most plant oils contain relatively little of the stuff. *But*, there are some important exceptions to this simple rule. Chicken, turkey, rabbit and oily fish like herring and mackerel have fats which are less saturated than other animal fats, and so provide useful alternatives in the diet. Whereas two plant oils, coconut oil and palm oil, are highly saturated. Indeed coconut oil makes meat and dairy fats seem almost saintly by comparison.

And polyunsaturates?

Many of the less saturated fats – like corn oil, soya oil, sunflower oil, safflower oil and fish oils – are 'high in polyunsaturates'. Unlike saturated fats, polyunsaturates do *not* increase blood cholesterol – indeed they may reduce it. So when it comes to cutting down fat, it's the mainly saturated fat that should go.

## A word about the cholesterol in your food

There's been so much talk about cholesterol these past few years that you'd be forgiven for thinking that it was the root of all evil. Certainly in America they've really taken cholesterol to heart. It's become such a big bogey there that you only have to whisper the word in the executive dining room and they all clutch their chests in fear and trepidation.

Cholesterol is not strictly speaking a fat, but it is a 'fat-like' substance. It is made naturally in our bodies, and in the bodies of all animals. In fact it is vital to the functioning of our cells, being a necessary constituent of cell membranes.

We make as much cholesterol as we need, and because we also eat a certain amount of cholesterol in our food, we automatically make adjustments to try to compensate for that. In this way the level of cholesterol in our bodies, and particularly in our blood, should remain fairly constant.

Unfortunately, this system can be upset

- by eating too much fat, particularly saturated fat, which seems to push up the cholesterol level in the blood
- by eating too much cholesterol in our food, so that the compensating system is overwhelmed and the blood cholesterol level goes up
- by having an inbuilt fault in the compensating system so that even moderate intakes of fat and cholesterol are enough to push up the blood cholesterol level.

As we've already mentioned, a high blood cholesterol level can be bad news for the heart, and so it pays to take steps to avoid that. That means either eating less saturated fat or cholesterol or both. Cholesterol is found in concentrated form in egg yolks, offal and shellfish. But most of the cholesterol the average person eats comes in meat and dairy foods because those are the main foods that come from animal sources which nearly all contain some cholesterol, whereas there is no cholesterol in food from plants.

Unless you happen to be an egg-freak, guzzling two or three a day (or more), your cholesterol intake in the form of egg yolks is unlikely to be making much difference to the total amount of cholesterol and saturated fat that you eat. Some experts have recommended that up to three or four eggs a week is sensible moderation. But it would be next to useless to make a token effort with eggs while the rest of your food is swimming in saturated fat.

And while we're on this subject, don't be fooled by labels on cooking oils and the like which say 'no cholesterol' or 'low cholesterol'. What they don't tell you is whether they are high or low in saturated fat, and that's much more important for most people.

### Where's the fat in the British diet?

27% comes from the meat products
13% from milk
13% from margarine
13% from cooking oils, lard, etc
12% from butter
6% from biscuits, cakes and pastries
5% from cheese and cream
3% from eggs
9% from other foods

## Fibre: is life rough enough for you?

Just about the biggest change in nutritional thinking over the past decade or so has been the realisation that what we used to dismiss as mere 'roughage' is actually a very important part of our diet indeed. Now rechristened 'dietary fibre', it is the one thing that most of us just aren't getting enough of.

Fibre. The very word conjures up pictures of sackcloth and ashes. Of self-denial and punishment. But what exactly is the stuff?

Fibre consists of the cell walls of plants – seeds, shoots, roots, leaves, flowers, fruits. It isn't one substance, but a complex mixture of many different substances, which vary greatly depending on what plant foods you eat. But they all have one thing in common – they are mostly not absorbed in the digestive tract. The mixture just passes clean through. And in doing so it provides the bowels with bulk or roughage, which actually smoothes the flow of food residue through the system. Far from being rough or stringy, it's a smooth, soft, water-absorbent gel. Perhaps 'smoothage' would be a better description of dietary fibre. In the last twenty years or so, observations around the world have pointed to a link between Western man's modern refined low fibre diet and several of the 'diseases of affluence' which afflict him – constipation, bowel diseases like diverticular disease and bowel cancer, gallstones, piles, varicose veins, appendicitis and, linked with being overweight, diabetes and heart disease. All were virtually unknown in industrialised countries in the middle of the last century, and they

18

are still rare in many developing countries where the diet is high in fibre. For instance, in rural Africa the average time taken for food to pass through the digestive system is about 36 hours. In Britain it varies from three days in young people to as long as two weeks in the elderly. Rural Africans eat four to five times more fibre than the average person in the UK. To put that in perspective, British vegetarians eat about twice the national average fibre intake. They also suffer less from bowel disorders like diverticular disease and irritable bowel syndrome. The likely reason is that fibre absorbs water; so with a high fibre diet, the stools are softer and more bulky. This not only speeds up transit time (things shift along a bit quicker) but also the smoothness of flow means that the bowels do not have to strain away, building up such high pressures.

About four out of ten Britons reckon they are constipated and about one person in five takes laxatives – five million pounds' worth every year. Laxatives aren't the answer of course. The best (and the most natural) way to break the logjam is for us all to eat more high fibre foods – more wholegrain (unrefined) cereal, such as wholemeal bread and wholewheat breakfast cereals; more unprocessed vegetables; more pulses, such as beans and peas; more fresh fruit and more nuts. And that applies just as much to those who don't regard themselves as constipated, because there are many other benefits of having a faster bowel transit time and lower bowel pressure.

Irritable bowel, a common disorder in young women causing colicky abdominal pains; diverticular disease, suffered by hundreds of thousands of middle-aged and elderly people, with sudden inflammation of the large bowel; cancer of the large bowel, second only to lung cancer as a cause of cancer deaths; piles (haemorrhoids), a very common and distressing ailment – all these conditions that are so much a part of the Western way of life (and in some cases death) are very rare in the Third World. Scientists are becoming increasingly convinced that these disorders can all be blamed, at least partly, on our sluggish high-pressure bowel action.

And that much more fibre in our food is the natural answer.

But, quite apart from all this bowel business, as everyone must know by now, *high fibre foods are the natural key to slim, fit, positive health*. Whole cereals, pulses, leafy and root vegetables, fruit and nuts, can provide a whole feast of essential nutrients without loading you down with concentrated calories, fat, sugar or salt. For the calories in a heaped tablespoon of sugar or a half-ounce pat of butter (or margarine) you could chew a thick slice of wholemeal bread, or nearly half a pound of peas. Indeed, in many ways high fibre foods are the antidote to our modern diet. We still have essentially the same bodies as Stone Age Man, with the same digestive system. Anthropological studies have revealed that humans evolved as omnivores, eating a mixture of plant and animal food, but with the great bulk of their diet coming from cereal seeds, fleshy roots, nut and fruit. Meat was usually just a rare treat if the hunters had been lucky that day.

Like all game, the meat that early Man sank his canines into was very lean and low in fat in comparison to today's overfed cattle and plumped-up pigs. There was salt in meat and, for those living near water, in fish; but otherwise salt was a rare commodity indeed. Sugar was found in fruit, roots and young shoots, diluted with plenty of fibre, the only really concentrated source widely available being honey.

Once you start to think of the sort of diet our digestive system evolved to deal with, and what we're forcing through it today, you can see why it is that so many of our modern illnesses are the sad result of living, and eating, in a world too far removed from nature.

## Where's the fibre in the British diet?

48% comes from vegetables
30% from cereals and bread
10% from fruit
12% from nuts etc

## Sweet talk about sugar and your health

What a seductive substance sugar is! Sweet delight! So tempting, so 'more-ish', almost addictive. Surely one of life's few harmless pleasures. How can a substance so pure be anything but positively healthy?

Certainly the sweet and sugar manufacturers would like you to believe that. They take such great pains to extol the virtues of sugar as a valuable source of energy, you might be tempted to think there is something special about it that somehow perks you up and acts as a sort of tonic. If only that were true.

Certainly sugar is a source of energy; but for 'energy' read 'calories', because make no mistake about it, they are precisely the same thing. Calories are simply measures of energy. Very few of us these days are short of calories. So it's not surprising that you never hear an advertisement say something like 'Nibble a NutKin for instant calories!'

Apart from its calories *there is absolutely nothing of any nutritional significance in sugar*. White or brown, it makes no difference; brown is no 'healthier' than white. Since virtually everything else you eat contains calories there is no need to eat any sugar at all. And that includes glucose as well as 'ordinary' sugar (sucrose). Although your body runs on glucose it can make all it needs from the great mixture of food you eat. And it keeps 'instant' reserves stored as glycogen in your liver and muscles.

We all know how nice sugar is . . . but how 'naughty' is it? Is it actually harmful to health?

As we've already said, being overweight, even less than a stone overweight, increases your risk of two particular health problems – high blood pressure and diabetes, both of which are linked to heart attacks and strokes.

If you tend to put on weight easily, then any high calorie food is bad news as far as your health is concerned. Sugar has no saving graces like useful fibre or vitamins. So, as every slimmer knows, if you want to lose weight without missing out on vital nutrients, sugar and sweet sugary things are best set aside for the occasional treat only.

But apart from the calories is sugar itself any threat to health?

Some scientific evidence suggests that eating very sugary food can put a sufficient strain on the body chemistry to increase the risk of diabetes, and gallstones even in slim people. But this effect is little more than a suspicion at this stage and further research needs to be done to verify it. On the other hand there is plenty of evidence that frequent eating or drinking of sugary things can lead to tooth decay.

The mouth contains bacteria which tend to gather in the nooks and crannies around the teeth. Food residue, including sugary food residue, tends to collect in the same places. The bacteria feed off the food residue, multiplying rapidly to form the cheesy deposit called plaque. As the sugary residue is fermented, the plaque becomes more acidic and soon starts to dissolve away the tooth enamel. This process lasts for up to an hour after the sugar has been taken. Once the enamel is perforated, a cavity will rapidly develop.

Eating or drinking sugar on more than three occasions during the course of the day gives rise to more than three hours of exposure to acid plaque. You can imagine the effect that can have on tooth enamel – not unlike the effect of acid rain on marble buildings. Of course the whole process of tooth decay is more complex than that, and many other factors are involved, but it does look as though the *more often* sugary things are in the mouth, the greater the likelihood of tooth decay. Fluoride in toothpaste, mouthwashes and drinking water undoubtedly helps to protect against this process. So too does regular careful brushing of teeth to remove plaque. But the crucial thing is to cut down the number of times sugary things are eaten or drunk, especially *between meals*. Soft drinks with sugar or glucose in, sweets, ices, biscuits, sugary snacks and tea or coffee with sugar added – all make an ideal breeding ground for acid plaque. The obvious answer is to cut right down on between-meal snacks, or switch to savoury nibbles that are safer for teeth.

Before we leave the subject of sugar, just one more point. Honey is a delicious and quite remarkable substance. Remarkable, that is, in its origin; just to think of all those bees buzzing in and out of all those flowers . . . No wonder it's been invested with almost magical qualities throughout the centuries. But the sad fact is that, just like sugar, honey has no nutrients in any significant amounts whatsoever. All it offers in abundance is calories.

## Salt and blood pressure

High blood pressure (or 'hypertension') isn't exactly a disease. It isn't even a symptom. Indeed you probably wouldn't know you had got high blood pressure until it either was discovered at a medical check-up or it caused a calamity. Perhaps a sudden stroke, with paralysis down one side of the body. Perhaps a heart attack or angina. Perhaps kidney failure. High blood pressure is the likely cause of many serious, life-threatening disorders, which all too often strike out of the blue because high blood pressure itself is symptomless.

Unfortunately it is a surprisingly common condition. The figures vary according to the precise definition of what constitutes 'high' blood pressure, but it is usually reckoned that about one adult in ten has a blood pressure high enough to need some action to correct it. This proportion rises to about one in four people in middle age.

What causes hypertension?

Sometimes it is caused by a malfunction of the kidneys or a gland, but in the great majority of cases it just happens for no obvious reason. The pressure of blood in the arteries very gradually creeps up over a period of months or years. The precise mechanism is only beginning to be understood, but it seems to be linked with the balance of sodium and potassium in the body. A fault in the system controlling this balance may eventually lead to high blood pressure. One possible way in which this control system may be upset or at least strained is by eating a diet which is too high in sodium. Experiments with animals and with human volunteers have shown that high sodium diets can push up the blood pressure. What's more, low sodium diets have been used successfully to lower the raised blood pressure of some hypertensive patients.

The main source of sodium in our diet is of course common salt. Whether it be table salt, cooking salt, sea salt or rock salt, it is all the same compound, sodium chloride. The British eat an awful lot of sodium chloride – on average about twelve grams a day. That's about two and a half teaspoonsful! It's also about fifteen or twenty times more than our bodies actually need, unless we happen to be working in particularly sweaty circumstances. And yet Britain is by no means at the top of the international salt-eating league. The Japanese eat even more salt, probably because so much of their diet is fish, brine pickles and salty soy sauce. Researchers have studied whole populations to see whether their average salt intake has any effect on their average blood pressure, and they have found that, broadly speaking, *high salt eaters have higher blood pressures than low salt eaters*. Indeed, salt intake and blood pressure seem to go hand in hand, and the more salt a population consumes per head, the more people have hypertension.

Does this mean then that the more salt you eat the more likely you are to get high blood pressure?

This has been difficult to prove clearly because people vary so much in their reaction to salt. Some blood pressures go right up; others hardly move. As more research is done, it's beginning to look as though about one person in five may be particularly susceptible to salt and run an extra risk of getting hypertension.

The snag is that there isn't an easy way of knowing whether you are one of these more vulnerable people. At present there is no simple screening test for salt sensitivity. The only clue comes from your family history. If your mother, father, brother or sister has had high blood pressure then there may be a family tendency to salt sensitivity and you may be next in line. In those circumstances it obviously makes sense to have your blood pressure checked by your family doctor.

Another important factor is your age. In countries where the average diet is quite high in salt, the older people become the more likely they are to develop high blood pressure. This effect of age on blood pressure is rarely found in low salt eating societies. In practical terms it means that if you are over thirty-five you would be wise to have your blood pressure checked regularly – say, every five years.

If for any reason your blood pressure is found to be significantly raised then you will probably have to have some sort of medication to bring it back down again to normal levels and keep it there.

In other words, you will usually have to take drugs for life.

Obviously all this is best avoided if possible. There are five main ways in which you might reduce your risk of developing hypertension: by not smoking, by taking regular exercise, by learning to cope with stress, and, as far as your diet is concerned, by avoiding being overweight and cutting down on salt.

## Where's the salt in the British diet?

33% is added in cooking and at the table
33% comes from cereals and bread
17% from meat and meat products
17% from all other foods

## Protein: the land of plenty

Protein malnutrition is virtually unheard of in Western nations.

On average we are eating about twice as much protein as we need. It is difficult for us to go short of protein and even children, adolescents and pregnant women, who need relatively more protein to build new tissue, will be well provided for by eating the sort of varied diet we advocate in this book. While it's true that meat is an excellent source of protein, a combination of cereals and pulses can provide protein which is just as good, much cheaper and without that unwanted hanger-on – saturated fat.

Incidentally, eating extra protein won't make you extra strong and beefy. Your body simply burns the surplus to produce calories – indeed protein contains more calories than carbohydrate does. So the chances are you'll just get extra big . . . where you don't want to be!

## Vitamins and minerals: goodies galore

Leaf through any of the women's magazines, or the new breed of health and fitness glossies, and you'll find page after page of advertisements extolling the virtues of multivitamin and mineral pills. It's very big business indeed. The advertisers go on about today's stresses, rushed meals, junk snacks and inadequate slimming diets, and offer their particular panacea in the shape of a rather expensive pill.

But is there any evidence that many of us are really going short of vitamins and minerals? And are pills the sensible answer?

In fact, cases of vitamin deficiency are very much a rarity in Western countries. According to the British National Food Survey, the average household's shopping basket contains a range of foods with vitamin and mineral levels way above the officially recommended daily requirements for each person. Getting enough vitamins and minerals is crucial to good health, but the fact is that 'enough' means very tiny quantities indeed. For instance, for Vitamin C (which is the vitamin we need the largest amount of) the recommended daily amount for adults is 30mg. That's less than you'll get from half an orange; or about as much as there is in the traditional 'two veg' of mashed potatoes and boiled cabbage.

Vitamin C and the B vitamins are the ones our bodies cannot store and which we therefore need in small quantities every day. They also happen to be the ones most easily destroyed by long storage, canning and cooking. For Vitamin C, for instance, this means that it's best to eat fruit and vegetables freshly picked and either raw or quickly and lightly cooked. Later on in this book we give some tips on how to choose and cook for healthier eating.

As to minerals, lack of iron in the diet can cause a common form of anaemia or 'thin' blood, particularly in women of childbearing age. But if you follow the advice in this book to eat more fresh fruit and vegetables, their vitamin C can help your body to absorb more than enough iron.

To return to the question of those vitamin and mineral supplements – if you eat a varied diet of the sort we describe in this book, you will be getting easily enough of the whole range of vitamins and minerals known to be necessary for good health. Taking extra vitamins and minerals will not be 'extra' good for you. Depending on the particular vitamin or mineral, your body either gets rid of the surplus in the urine or shoves it aside in the body stores.

What a waste of hard-earned money!

# The NACNE targets: nutritional goals for the year 2000

Take a look at most other books on healthy eating and you'll find that they all say roughly the same things: *eat less fat, eat less sugar, eat less salt and eat plenty of fibre.*

It's all very well being told to eat 'less' of this or 'more' of that or 'plenty' of the other. But HOW MUCH less? And HOW MUCH more? And HOW MUCH is meant by plenty?

Nutritional advice has been so vague for so long that people can hardly be blamed for not bothering to change their eating habits for fear of getting the balance all wrong and going down with beri-beri or some such deficiency disorder. What is needed is a set of fairly precise targets to aim at: some pretty firm figures giving the desirable quantities of the most critical components in our everyday diet – fat, fibre, sugar and salt.

There have been tables and target figures published in the past. But these have been a hangover from the days when malnutrition was a real threat and so their main purpose has been to provide figures for the MINIMUM daily amounts of vital nutrients and calories required for health.

These minimum daily requirements are a useful guide for those catering for large numbers of people but are of little use as a nutritional guide for individuals when they are choosing what to eat.

What most people need are target figures giving the MAXIMUM for the three 'baddies' in their food:

- fat (particularly *saturated* fat)
- sugar (mostly sucrose)
- salt (particularly the sodium part of it)

The only MINIMUM that matters for most people these days is for the now famous 'goody':

- fibre (from a mixture of cereals, pulses, fruit and vegetables)

By giving precise targets for all these food elements the NACNE

Report has broken new ground. And it's these targets that form the basis of Diet 2000.

The NACNE targets are intended for the average adult to have achieved by the year 2000. The reason why NACNE has proposed this long delay is to give the agriculture and food industries time to make the necessary changes to be able to cater for the massive switch in eating habits.

But you don't have to worry too much about how the farmers and food suppliers will cope. That's not your problem. And anyway, take our word for it, they'll manage all right. There's nothing like a new surge of consumer demand for persuading the food barons to rethink their product lines and start selling what people want. So you don't have to wait until the end of the century to start eating for health. It could be too late by then. The time to switch to the new targets is NOW.

Because the NACNE targets are designed for the average adult they will have to be adjusted to suit you or the various members of your family. Later in the book we show you how to make the necessary allowances for your age, sex, activity level and body weight using our unique Diet 2000 Personal Eating Planner on page 31.

But first here are the key targets in the original NACNE-type language, followed by our translation for those who wouldn't know a fatty acid if it hit them between the eyes.

- **Energy intake should be appropriate for maintaining optimal body weight for height and sex, with adequate exercise.** This means that if you have a tendency to put on weight easily you should try to keep within the 'desirable' weight range for your height (see page 13) by avoiding too much high calorie food and taking regular moderately vigorous exercise (yes, it makes sense to think of exercise as part of your Diet 2000). See the Personal Eating Planner on page 31.
- **Fat intake should be on average 30 per cent of total energy intake.** This means that the total amount of fat in your food should provide no more than thirty per cent of all the calories you eat and drink (including alcohol). At the moment the fat in the average person's diet supplies about thirty-eight per cent of the total calorie intake. In other words, out of every five calories you eat or drink, two come from fat. The NACNE target means the

average person should aim to *cut total fat by nearly a quarter*. In the pages that follow we tell you how that reduction can be achieved.

- **Saturated fatty acid intake should be on average 10 per cent of total energy intake.** This means that the saturated fat in your food (mainly in the form of dairy produce and meat, but also in the form of certain plant oils) should provide no more than 10 per cent of all the calories you eat and drink (including alcohol). At the moment saturated fat supplies about 18 per cent of the average person's calories, so the NACNE target means *cutting saturated fat by nearly half*. In Diet 2000 we tell you how.

- **Average sucrose intake should be reduced to 20 kg per head per year.** This means that the average person should reduce their consumption of sugar by nearly half, from the current intake of 38 kg per head per year to 20 kg. That's from just over 100 g (4 oz) a day to just over 50 g. Or from about 8 tablespoonsfuls to about 4, of which no more than half should be in the form of between-meal sweets, snacks and sugared drinks. Remember that this is a *maximum* average intake, so if you usually eat less than an average 50 g of sugar a day then don't be tempted to increase it. Diet 2000 will help you find out how much sugar you're eating and if necessary cut down.

- **Average salt intake should fall by 3 g per head per day.** It is currently about 12 g per head per day, so 3 g represents a 25 per cent cut, down from about 2½ teaspoonsful to less than 2. Again this is a *maximum* so if you're currently eating less than 9 g of salt a day, don't feel you should be making up your losses. Diet 2000 will help you keep tabs on the salt in your food.

- **Fibre intake should increase on average from 20 g to 30 g per head per day.** This means the average person should be eating half as much again of fibre. Remember the 30 g is a *minimum* average figure. So if you're already eating more than that, keep chewing! In Diet 2000 you'll find out how to reap all that extra fibre.

As well as these main proposals NACNE recommends that our average alcohol intake should fall to at most 4 per cent of our total calories. That's an average of 20 g a day maximum – which is less than one pint of beer or two glasses of wine. Maximum, remember!

As far as protein is concerned NACNE recommends no change. We are getting enough as it is. Indeed we're getting about twice as much as we need on average.

NACNE recommends that we need not concern ourselves with cholesterol in our food, providing we follow the recommendations for fats.

As for vitamins and minerals, NACNE says that the recommendations outlined above would automatically increase their intake to well above the recommended daily allowances. In other words, with Diet 2000 vitamins and minerals take care of themselves.

So those are the famous NACNE recommendations stripped to the bare bones.

But what do they mean as far as you are concerned?

And what will happen to your food?

Next, in Part Two, we look at how you can adapt the NACNE targets to suit your individual needs.

# Part Two:
# Diet 2000 in action

## The Diet 2000 Personal Eating Planner: how to fix your own targets for fat, sugar, salt and fibre

The NACNE recommendations are designed as goals for the 'average' person.

But everybody's different.

Male or female, young or old, active or inactive, fat or thin, and with all the possibilities in between – surely there's no such creature as the average person.

So where do you fit into the scheme of things? And how can you make the necessary adjustments to the NACNE targets so that they are right for you?

That's where the Diet 2000 Personal Eating Planner comes in.

We believe you'll find it the simplest way yet devised to work out

- how much fat, fibre, sugar and salt there is in the food you are eating at the moment
- how much you should be eating, according to your age, sex, activity level and body weight
- how to translate that into actual items of food so that you know what changes you need to make to your diet to stay slimmer and live longer.

Then, when you know what you're aiming at, we take you shopping to help you choose the Diet 2000 balance of foods; we give you a hand in the kitchen with a few tips to keep you on your Diet 2000 target; and we offer you a range of menus and recipes to show you how, with Diet 2000, you can make meals that are not just waistline-trimming and health-enhancing – but mouthwatering as well!

The Diet 2000 Personal Eating Planner is a unique step-by-step system using simple symbols to guide you to a healthy diet. What's more it sets targets based on your personal energy requirements – so you can stay slim without the need to count a single calorie! First you need to look very closely indeed at what you're eating, day by

31

day; and by using our Diet 2000 Food Score Tables, to find out how much fat, fibre, sugar and salt you are eating at the moment. For fibre, sugar and salt you can then check straight away with the NACNE targets to see how well (or badly!) you compare. But for fat your target has to be based on your total energy intake, and to do that, we've devised a simple chart which takes into account your age, sex, physical activity level and body weight. As you'll see, we've done all the complicated calculations for you and the chart gives you a target for fat.

By comparing your scores with your targets for the fat, fibre, sugar and salt in your food, you'll be able to see how much needs changing. And by looking through the Food Score Tables and following our general advice on healthy eating you'll soon know how to go about it.

OK, so much for theory – let's get on with it. But before we do, just a few words about our simple symbol scoring system for the fat, fibre, sugar and salt in food.

As you know there are plenty of other books around which give exhaustive (and exhausting!) lists of foods together with the number of 'calories per 100 g' (whatever that is!) or the number of 'grams of fibre per oz' or the percentage of this and that. We know that many people find the long lists of numbers rather difficult to handle, and that it's not easy to see how different foods compare for, let's say, fat and salt, or sugar and fibre, or any other combination.

We believe our food scoring system using symbols rather than numbers makes it all much simpler, and much easier to see at a glance, what's in what.

To understand the system all you have to know is that:

- the symbol for fat is ♠
- the symbol for fibre is ✿
- the symbol for sugar is ▨
- the symbol for salt is ◊

Right. Here we go with the step-by-step Diet 2000 Personal Eating Planner.

## Step 1: Look hard at what you're eating

Most people – even people who are quite fussy about their food – have only a vague idea as to what's really in the stuff they shovel down their throats. And they rarely stop to think *why* they chose those particular things. Was it habit? Was it price? Was it convenience? Or, dare we mention it, was it for health?

Now is the time to take a very close look at what you're eating and why. It means a bit of homework, and perhaps some memory-jogging, but you'll find it's worth the effort.

Take a look at the chart below. As you can see, it's a list of a

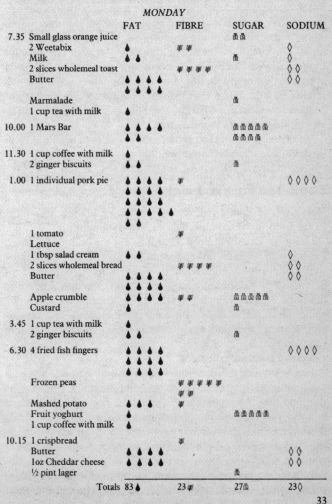

### MONDAY

| Time | | FAT | FIBRE | SUGAR | SODIUM |
|---|---|---|---|---|---|
| 7.35 | Small glass orange juice | | | ●●(sugar ×2) | |
| | 2 Weetabix | | ×2 | | ◇ |
| | Milk | ●● | | ×1 | ◇ |
| | 2 slices wholemeal toast | | ×4 | | ◇◇ |
| | Butter | ●●●● ●●●● | | | ◇◇ |
| | Marmalade | | | ×1 | |
| | 1 cup tea with milk | ● | | | |
| 10.00 | 1 Mars Bar | ●●●● ●● | | ×4 ×4 | |
| 11.30 | 1 cup coffee with milk | ● | | | |
| | 2 ginger biscuits | ●● | | ×1 | |
| 1.00 | 1 individual pork pie | ●●●● ●●●● ●●●● ●● | ×1 | | ◇◇◇◇ |
| | 1 tomato | | ×1 | | |
| | Lettuce | | | | |
| | 1 tbsp salad cream | ●● | | | ◇ |
| | 2 slices wholemeal bread | | ×4 | | ◇◇ |
| | Butter | ●●●● | | | ◇◇ |
| | Apple crumble | ●●●● | ×2 | ×4 | |
| | Custard | ● | | ×1 | |
| 3.45 | 1 cup tea with milk | ● | | | |
| | 2 ginger biscuits | ●● | | ×1 | |
| 6.30 | 4 fried fish fingers | ●●●● ●●●● ●●●● | | | ◇◇◇◇ |
| | Frozen peas | | ×6 | | |
| | Mashed potato | ●●● | | | |
| | Fruit yoghurt | ● | | ×4 | |
| | 1 cup coffee with milk | ● | | | |
| 10.15 | 1 crispbread | | ×1 | | |
| | Butter | ●●●● | | | ◇◇ |
| | 1oz Cheddar cheese | ●●●● | | | ◇◇ |
| | ½ pint lager | | | ×1 | |
| | **Totals** | **83 ●** | **23 ×** | **27 sugar** | **23 ◇** |

33

typical day's food and drink for one person. We suggest you fill in a chart like this, noting everything that passes your lips, every day for a whole week – most people's eating habits tend to follow a weekly pattern. It's easiest to use ruled sheets of paper and start each day on a new sheet. You should put down every single item, food or drink, including snacks and sweets, and make a note of the time of day and the approximate quantity. Remember it must include everything, from the moment you wake up in the morning, to the last thing at night. The quantities don't have to be exact – this isn't the Spanish Inquisition – just the number of portions or pieces or, if you're good at it, a guess for the weight. Leave the fat, fibre, sugar and salt scoring till later. If you can't manage those for a whole week, three or four days including Saturday and Sunday should give you a fair idea of what's going down the hatch.

Incidentally, if you can persuade the rest of the family to join in this exercise, so much the merrier.

## Step 2: The day of reckoning

When you've completed your diary, and you've a few quiet moments to spare, sit yourself down for some totting up.

Using the Diet 2000 Food Score Table at the back of the book, look up each item and make a note in the diary of what it scores for the four key constituents: fat, fibre, sugar and salt (if the exact item is not listed, choose the nearest equivalent). As you see, we've devised a unique symbol system to make it really easy to see at a glance how your food is balancing out. We suggest you count the symbol scores and mark the number in the appropriate column in your diary.

Now sit back and take stock.

Just by keeping the diary you will have already learned a lot about your eating habits, perhaps even the odd little shock revelation as the food lists show you where the hidden fat, sugar and salt is lurking. You will probably already have a shrewd idea of which of those three 'baddies' you have overdosed on. But what you really need to know is how much. And how far short of your fibre target you are.

So add up the symbols in each of the four columns – fat, fibre, sugar and salt – and fill in the table for each day. Then, just for good measure, add up the totals for the whole week and divide by seven to get the daily average. Now at last you're ready to compare your present eating scores with your own personal Diet 2000 targets.

## Step 3: Setting your own targets

### Your fat target

Take a look at the NACNE targets again and you'll see that, while they give straightforward fixed amounts for the average intake of fibre, sugar and salt, the target for fat is linked to total energy (calorie) intake.

This is because fat is a major source of calories, and to give a fixed figure without reference to the overall calorie requirements would be quite unrealistic. Be that as it may, you need to know just how much fat you should be eating for *you*, in terms you can understand, like pats of butter and lamb chops.

So here is your Diet 2000 Fat Target Indicator.

And here's how to use it:

i)   Decide on your *age* and *sex* (no comment!).
ii)  Estimate your habitual *activity level*. 'Moderately active' means that you carry out any moderately vigorous activity (enough to make you a bit puffed) for about twenty to thirty minutes at a time, two or three times a week. Anything from brisk walking to aerobics, or from bedmaking to digging. Less than that is 'sedentary'; more is 'very active'.
iii) Check your *weight*. Turn to the height/weight charts on page 13 and find out just how desirable you are – weightwise. If you are above the desirable range for your height, i.e., in the 'overweight' or 'obese' brackets, you can adjust your personal target so that Diet 2000 helps you slim . . . and helps you stay there.

Now you can work out your personal target in terms of fat symbols, ( ◊ ) according to your age, sex and activity. The Indicator gives the daily targets for normal-weight adults.

You'll notice that it doesn't include targets for children. This is because children grow at such different rates at different ages that it is impossible to summarise all the variations in their energy requirements in a simple table like this. But you can assume that their fat target should not exceed that for moderately active young adults of the same sex. And of course all the general principles of Diet 2000 which we go into later apply just as much to them. Above all, Diet 2000 is about your whole family's eating.

## THE DIET 2000 FAT TARGET INDICATOR

| | Age | Sedentary | Activity level Moderately | Very |
|---|---|---|---|---|
| Men | 18–34 | 40 | 50 | 55 |
| | 35–64 | 40 | 45 | 55 |
| | 65+ | 40 | 45 | — |
| Women | 18–54 | 35 | 35 | 40 |
| | 55+ | 30 | 30 | — |
| | Pregnant | — | 40 | — |
| | Lactating | — | 45 | — |

*Note*

This table indicates the daily target of fat symbols for various categories of people, according to their age, sex and activity level.

The table is based on the Department of Health's Recommended Daily Amounts of Food Energy (1979) and the NACNE target for total fat.

So, now you have a daily fat target to compare with your food diary scores. Remember it's very much an average figure. Your daily intake of fat will probably vary greatly from day to day, especially at weekends, so it's best to compare your target with your average daily fat score. Also, because it's based on average figures for the population at large, you may feel that it's too generous for you; in which case reduce your target by five.

## How to lose weight with Diet 2000

If you are 'overweight' you should aim for 10 fat symbols less than the number indicated. For the average person this should give a weight loss of about 1lb a week.

If you are 'obese' you should aim for 15 fat symbols less than the number indicated, giving the average person a weight loss of about 1½lb a week.

So, to give you an example.

Let's say you're a 32-year-old mother of three young children who keep you on your toes all day, and that you do twice-weekly aerobics because you're a bit overweight.

You're likely to be in the 'very active' bracket; and that would give you a target for your age and sex of 40 fat symbols. But you've got to get your weight down, so subtract 10 from the 40, leaving you a daily target of 30 fat symbols.

As you approach your desirable weight you can gradually increase your fat target until you reach the standard for your age, sex and activity level.

So as you see, Diet 2000 is not only a staying slim diet – it's also a *getting* slim diet. In fact you can lose as much weight with it as with any other low fat, high fibre diet. But the great advantage of Diet 2000 is that once you've lost weight you're much more likely to stay that way. Why? Because you are not just 'on a diet'. Instead you will have made the principles embodied in Diet 2000 part of your normal everyday life.

### *Your fibre target*

Compared with all the fiddling with fat, your fibre target is a very simple matter indeed. The NACNE recommendation was for the average person to eat 30g a day. Fortunately no special allowances have to be made for people of different ages, etc., except to say that slimmers and people over thirty-five should, if anything, aim rather higher than this, up to 40g.

Translated into the Diet 2000 symbol system, younger people should set themselves a target of 15 fibre symbols (🌾) a day. Slimmers and older people, a target of 20. This is an average daily target; there'll be days when you eat more, and others when you eat less.

### *Your sugar limit*

Notice we've called this a 'limit' rather than a target because, as we said on page 21, cutting sugar intake down to a minimum will do no harm and may do much good.

According to NACNE the average person should be limited to 20kg a year of sucrose ('ordinary' sugar). That works out at an average of 55g a day, which is about 11 level teaspoonsful. Of course, that includes all the 'hidden' sugar in your food as well as the stuff you spoon into your tea or coffee. With the Diet 2000 symbol system your limit is 11 sugar symbols (🍬) daily. However, that's an average limit; so in practice if you go over the limit one day, you should aim under it (by at least the same amount) the next. What's more, according to NACNE, no more than half the sugar you eat should come from between-meal snacks and drinks. So it's a maximum of five of your sugar symbols from these. And remember, the less sugar you eat, the more starchy high fibre food you're allowed.

## Your salt limit

NACNE recommends that the average person should be limited to 9g a day; that's just under 2 teaspoonsful. That includes all the hidden salt in your food as well as what's shaken on it in cooking and eating. It's an average figure; some days you'll eat more, others less. People with high blood pressure (themselves, or in the family) should try to eat less than 9g a day.

The Diet 2000 limit for salt is 15 salt symbols (◊) a day. In fact this represents not only salt (sodium chloride) but also other forms of sodium such as baking soda, and monosodium glutamate. However, these other forms amount to less than one symbol a day. As with all the Diet 2000 targets and limits, the 15 salt symbols is an *average* daily figure. Modest fluctuation from day to day is quite OK.

## Step 4: How do you compare?

So now you know your daily targets for fat, fibre, sugar and salt, the next step is to compare these with your daily totals in your food diary. You could check with each day separately or with the average daily totals for the whole week.

How near or how far are you? Well over the top for fat?
Rather lacking in fibre?
Too tempted by sugar?
Addicted to salt?

The point of all this symbol counting is to see just how, and how much, you need to change your ways to be right by NACNE and improve your chances of a longer healthier life. The symbols are not just symbolic! They give you an easy way of making the necessary adjustments to your present diet.

So count the number of symbols that stand between you and the Diet 2000 targets and draw up your 'action list'. Here's a typical example:

- Cut fat by 10 symbols a day.
- Increase fibre by 5 symbols a day, at least.
- Reduce sugar by 11 symbols a day, especially in the form of between-meal sweets, snacks and sugary drinks.
- Reduce salt by 5 symbols a day.

Now in case you're wondering what to do about such other things in your food as starch (complex carbohydrate), protein, vitamins, minerals and trace elements, let's just quickly deal with them now.

*Protein* NACNE recommends no change for the average person. This means you carry on eating your 50-80g protein a day, 11 per cent of your total calorie intake (yes, even meat protein gives you calories!), which for the average person is equivalent to an 8oz sirloin steak. Please note, we're not suggesting that you actually eat a sirloin steak every day, far from it. In fact, with Diet 2000 much more of your protein will come from cereal foods like bread, breakfast cereals, rice and pasta, pulses like beans and peas; and vegetables.

*Vitamins, minerals and trace elements* For healthy people on a varied diet there is no shortage of these. Diet 2000 provides them all in abundance.

*Complex carbohydrate (starch)* Gone are the days when starchy foods were thought to be particularly fattening. *Unrefined* starchy foods are good because they come wrapped in fibre and laced with vitamins and minerals. The NACNE recommendations mean that over half (55 per cent) of your calories should come from carbohydrate, nearly all of which should be starch rather than sugar. So again it's bread, potatoes, rice, pasta, starchy vegetables and pulses. As you must have gathered by now, with Diet 2000 you'll be eating much more of these good things and on page 44 we show you how to plan your portions so that you get a healthy, wholesome and tasty variety of them.

Now, at last, it's time to put all the theory and mathematics behind you and to start thinking in terms of ordinary items of everyday food. This is where the Diet 2000 Food Scores come into play again. Study the lists and look at your diary and see which foods you could swap around to improve your eating. How are you going to lose 10 fat symbols? Eat less red meats and more chicken and fish instead? Less fried food? Less spread on your bread? Where are 5 fibre symbols going to come from? More wholemeat breakfast cereal? More wholemeal bread? Bigger portions of vegetables? Which 11 sugar symbols should go? The ones between meals certainly, but sweets? biscuits? sugar in your coffee?

And how to shake off the salt, all 5 symbols of it? Fewer packet soups? Less in cooking and at table?

The Diet 2000 eating plan with its symbol system was not intended to turn eating into a ghastly game of snakes and ladders. The last thing we want is for you to become obsessed with counting symbols here, there and everywhere. Eating is meant to be enjoyable. And we designed our system to help you relish your food in the knowledge that it isn't harming your health.

So once you've got a good idea of how much you need to change your eating, and what's in the various foods, you can push all those symbols right to the back of your mind, for reference only, and start planning, buying, cooking and eating the real thing . . . scrumptious, mouthwatering meals.

# Putting Diet 2000 to work

Now it's time to put Diet 2000 to work for you and your family, by bearing its simple guidelines in mind whenever you write a shopping list, reach for the frying pan or munch your rhubarb crunch.

And to help you along, in this last section of the book we offer our tips on how to choose, prepare and cook your food so that you keep well within your Diet 2000 targets while at the same time indulging yourself with delicious dishes made from our Diet 2000 recipes.

## How to use the Diet 2000 system to plan your eating

Before you rush out to the supermarket clutching your well-thumbed copy of Diet 2000, determined to revolutionise your eating habits, it's worth just sitting and thinking for a moment, and deciding what you and your family would usually want to eat over the next day or two, or week or two. The whole idea of Diet 2000 is that it's not just a five-minute-wonder diet to be tried out for a while to make you feel good or at least self-righteous. It's meant to be a way of eating for life – a diet to stick with and stay alive with.

So you, and your family, should be introduced to it gradually, in easy stages, a little change here and there.

Take sugar and salt for instance. They are both very strong, very 'addictive' tastes; and a liking for them is something most people have from a very early age. Unfortunately we're eating them both in potentially harmful quantities, and so we'd be wise to cut down. If you've ever tried to do that with either of them you'll know that the way to succeed is very gradually to wean yourself off by using smaller and smaller quantities over a period of a few weeks.

The same sort of approach can be applied to cutting down on saturated fat or eating more high fibre foods. Softly, softly – so that spouse and children hardly notice the quiet revolution under their noses.

So decide what change you are going to make this first week and plan your meals and your shopping accordingly. You might for instance feel that a relatively simple and painless change would be to eat a bowl of wholegrain breakfast cereal every morning. That's certainly a good start towards building up your fibre intake. We would suggest you choose a cereal which is not too salty or sugary, so take a look at the cereal section of the Diet 2000 Food Score Table on page 121, or compare cereals by studying the nutritional details on the packets.

You may decide to make some progress on the fat front by changing to semi-skimmed milk instead of your usual silver-top (or, heaven forbid, gold-top). Again that is a useful move (to see how useful turn to our chart on the fat content of milky things on page 53). Perhaps the easiest change to start with is to eat more fresh fruit and raw vegetables. After all this is *more* of something rather than less, so it's likely to be a popular move.

Other contenders for early action are: switching to wholemeal bread, cooking fewer fried meals, changing to chicken or fish more often, and eating a healthier snack rather than the mid-morning and mid-afternoon biscuits. Remember, we're not suggesting you make all these changes straight away. Just start with one or two and when you're used to the new arrangement slip in another one, and so on.

Another way to drift gently into Diet 2000 is to try one or two of our recipes each week and steadily build up a repertoire of wholesome healthy dishes. Or you could base one of this week's suppers on a menu from our season-by-season suggestions.

It's up to you how you go about changing to Diet 2000 – little by little or, if you're a revolutionary by nature, in one fell swoop. But the important thing is to make a start *now* . . . and think ahead.

*Will it be expensive?*

Short answer: NO . . . and if anything rather cheaper.

A glance through the Food Score Table will show you that a shift away from red meats towards chicken, fish and non-meat meals is likely to reduce fat intake. It's also likely to reduce the cost. Cereals are cheap.

Fruit and vegetables in season are cheap. Dried pulses are cheap.

On the other hand packaged 'convenience' foods and made-up meals are relatively expensive; so too are fatty salty snacks and sweets. So by buying fewer of these you'll be saving money. And by looking for new ways to eat the food you have in stock, including left-overs, you can keep costs down.

*Will it be too fiddly?*

Because you'll be moving away from tinned and packeted convenience foods towards dishes you prepare and cook yourself from the raw materials, you may think the whole business will be just too *in*convenient.

Obviously some extra effort is involved, but a look at our recipes will show you that it isn't too irksome. And if you have a freezer or freezing compartment in your fridge, you can prepare many of your meals in advance when you've got some time to spare. All you have to do then is remember to defrost each dish before you need it. In other words, you can make your own convenience foods.

*Will it be boring?*

No, not at all. Flick through our recipes. You'll see they're anything but boring. There's no less variety than in your present eating habits – after all you're not being asked to cut anything out completely, merely to cut down on some things. And the chances are you'll be enjoying some foods you don't often have, as you pick from the wide range of cereals, pulses, vegetables and fruit available, and you use lots of different herbs.

Diet 2000 is a diet you can live with because you can eat what you like. Maybe not as much as you like. Nor as often as like. But nevertheless what you like.

If you really fancy bacon and eggs on fried bread, or crave a chocolate éclair or two, that's just fine as long as you remember to take out an equal amount of fat and sugar from somewhere else in your week's eating so that you meet the Diet 2000 targets overall for the week.

Other diets are rigid with taboos – none of this, don't touch that. But Diet 2000 is a flexible eating plan. So don't expect every single meal to be in line with your targets. Nor every day necessarily. As long as the overall pattern for the week does work out well.

So make your plans with that general principle in mind – and give yourself and your family a few treats.

When you've made some changes and think you've probably got things about right, try keeping a food diary again and scoring it to see if you have reached your goals for fat, fibre, sugar and salt.

## Filling gaps

If you follow Diet 2000, far fewer of the calories in your food will come from fat. Instead a greater proportion will come from carbohydrates. And since you will also be eating less sugar, which is of course a 'simple' carbohydrate, the end result is that over half of your calories will be derived from so-called 'complex' carbohydrates, found mainly in starchy foods of plant origin – many of which are excellent sources of fibre.

But how do you decide on the right combination of low fat, mainly carbohydrate foods to get a good balance of calories, fibre and other nutrients? And how do you tailor the choice to suit your particular energy requirements? (And your appetite!)

One way is to use our Diet 2000 Fill-up Formula (below). All you do is find your Personal Fat Target in the left-hand column, and run your finger across the page to see how many standard portions from each main fill-up category you should eat each day.

### THE DIET 2000 DAILY FILL-UP FORMULA

| Your fat target | Number of portions* per day | | | | | |
|---|---|---|---|---|---|---|
| | Bread | Cereals | Starchy Veg | Leafy Veg | Fruit | Starchy Filler |
| 15 | 2 | 1 | 1 | 1 | 2 | 1 |
| 20 | 3 | 1 | 1 | 1 | 2 | 1 |
| 25 | 4 | 1 | 2 | 2 | 3 | 1 |
| 30 | 5 | 1 | 2 | 3 | 4 | 1 |
| 35 | 6 | 1 | 3 | 3 | 4 | 1 |
| 40 | 7 | 1 | 3 | 3 | 5 | 2 |
| 45 | 8 | 1 | 3 | 3 | 5 | 2 |
| 50 | 8 | 1 | 4 | 3 | 6 | 2 |
| 55 | 8 | 1 | 4 | 3 | 6 | 3 |

*Portion sizes are as detailed in the Food Score Table.

We suggest you use this chart when planning your menus to help you decide how many portions in the various 'fill-up' categories to eat each day, based on your overall energy requirements.

Of course this isn't all you will be eating; it's just the filling things to complement your main dishes.

To give an example: if you are a 45 fat-symbols-a-day person, you could eat eight slices of bread (preferably wholemeal), one serving of breakfast cereal (preferably wholegrain), three portions of any starchy vegetables (e.g. beans, peas, lentils, carrots, parsnips, beetroot, etc.), three portions of any leafy vegetables (e.g. spinach, broccoli, spring greens, brussels sprouts, cauliflower, cabbage, celery, lettuce, etc.), five portions of any fruit and two portions of starchy 'filler' (e.g. potato, rice or pasta) or one double-sized portion.

When choosing any particular item of food, check its *fibre* score in our Food Score Table at the back of the book. Aim for a daily total of not less than 15 fibre symbols.

# Setting a new pattern

When it comes to food most of us are very much creatures of habit. We get into a pattern of eating which seems to suit us, or our lifestyle, and we deviate very little from it. Maybe we usually have tea and toast for breakfast, or sandwiches for our midday meal, or a fry-up every evening. For some people no day's complete without a hot meal, and no meal's complete without meat, and no meat's complete without lots of brown gravy. Food is a great comforter, and habits are cosy.

For most people Diet 2000 will mean setting a new pattern to their day's eating, but if it's done carefully there's no reason why the new habits shouldn't be just as cosy as before.

Take breakfast, for instance.

As you'll see from our Fill-up Formula we suggest you have a portion of breakfast cereal every day (except perhaps on Saturday or Sunday for a change). The cereal should be wholegrain or whole-wheat to get all the fibre and protein, so check our Food Score Table or the nutritional details on the packet and watch out for added sugar and salt. Skimmed or semi-skimmed milk will help to keep your fat intake low, or use unsweetened fruit juice. You could slice some fresh fruit on it or scatter some mixed dried fruits. Don't forget porridge and muesli are excellent alternatives. If you think breakfasts are boring, take a look at some of the good ideas in our menu selection.

And if you haven't got the time or the stomach for cereal in the mornings, have some as a snack at night instead.

Whether you eat your main meal at midday or in the evening, and what it consists of, is again partly a question of habit and partly dependent on the time you want to spend choosing or preparing it. It's often lack of time that makes us fall back on the pre-cooked packaged convenience foods that are so often high in fat, sugar or salt, and low in fibre. But even when time is short we *can* eat in a healthier (and cheaper) way by basing at least one meal a day on bread and salad or fruit (e.g. a sandwich or roll). The choices will depend on the season, to get best value for money. The salad should preferably contain a starchy veg (e.g. carrots or sweetcorn) or a filler (e.g. potato or rice). There is nothing nutritionally superior about a hot meal – it won't do you any more good than a cold one – but it can certainly warm the spirit on a dull and miserable day. Soups are a fairly quick and easy way to do just that, and can be based on starchy or leafy vegetables. Again, bread is the natural accompaniment. We've included a number of satisfying soup recipes in our menu selection. Main meals can obviously be rather more elaborate if you have more time at your disposal. But more elaborate doesn't have to mean less healthy. And healthy doesn't have to mean dreary, as you'll soon discover.

## At the shops: how to choose food for the best of health

Here you are among the convenience foods and cream cakes, the bacon and biscuits, the pork pies and pastries. You are enticed by advertising, seduced by packaging and lulled into a reverie by the supermarket muzak. Yet it is now that you have to make some important decisions. You have to take home a healthy week's shopping.

To help you through this jungle we suggest you follow our Diet 2000 Five-Point Shopping Code:

1 **Be prepared**

Try to plan what you're going to eat, and make a list. Try also to be conscious of your Diet 2000 targets and get a feel for the symbol scores of the foods you are likely to be choosing. We're not suggesting you take your pocket calculator along with you but it helps to know what quantities of the various things you intend to buy. Imagine that your shopping basket will have to pass the 'NACNE Test'. Another advantage of planning is that it reduces the temptation to buy on impulse!

2 **Go it alone**

If you can, shop on your own. For one thing there will be less pressure on you to buy treats and pacifiers. And it also gives you a chance to concentrate a bit more on making the right choices. It's so much easier to get into the new diet if you've got time to linger among the fruit and vegetables, browse among the breads and hover over the wholefoods.

47

### 3 Shop around

This obviously makes good sense whatever you're eating. With Diet 2000 you'll be going much more for fresh fruit and vegetables in season, and wholefood alternatives. Most supermarkets stock all these items but you may find a small shop nearby that can beat them for prices.

### 4 Look at labels

Most labels now list the ingredients in descending order of weight, i.e. the main ingredient comes first. So watch out for foods which have near the top of the list sugar, sucrose, dextrose or glucose; salt, sodium or brine; suet, edible oil, vegetable oil or any other form of fat. Unfortunately, food manufacturers are not obliged at present to state *how much* fat, sugar or salt is in their product. And as for saturated fat, they don't even have to mention it. Hopefully this soon will be mandatory. Some foods, however, like cereals, have fairly informative labels, with a list of quantities stated which usually include fibre. Look for 'wholegrain' and 'wholewheat' products, fruits canned in 'natural juice', and vegetables canned without added salt.

### 5 Make demands

Use your consumer voice. If the shop doesn't stock the sort of food you want, put some pressure on the shopkeeper or supermarket manager. If enough people like you ask for it, it will appear like magic in no time at all. There's nothing like consumer demand for getting the food trade to react.

So, with this Five-Point Shopping Code in mind, let's wander round and make a few observations.

Starting at the bakery . . .

## *Your daily bread*

With Diet 2000 the humble loaf rises to new importance as bread becomes a bigger part of your everyday eating.

Bread is a major source of fibre in the average person's diet and, as more and more people switch to brown and wholemeal, it is rapidly becoming their number one fibre provider. Bread also gives you complex carbohydrate, protein, calcium, iron and vitamins; so it's a mistake to think of it as mere stodge, or packing material for a slice of ham. Bread has been a staple in the Western diet for centuries, but its consumption has been declining in recent years. This is no doubt partly because many people still regard it as 'starch' or 'carbohydrate', with nothing much else of nutritional value. Weight-conscious people in particular still tend to look on bread, and potatoes for that matter, as little more than sheer calories. How wrong they are!

Doctors and nutritionists the world over are now recognising the true value of bread in our diet. Not only is it a useful and inexpensive form of protein, vitamins and minerals, but also its complex carbohydrates and dietary fibre are a much healthier alternative to the fatty and sugary things we eat. The Royal College of Physicians in two recent reports, one on fibre, the other on obesity, has come out strongly in favour of a move back to fibre-rich starchy foods like bread, cereals and vegetables – for slimmers as well as everyone else.

So back to bread it is, then.

But before you reach for the packet of thin-sliced white . . . a few important points to bear in mind.

● First, there's bread . . . and bread. Many different types, with different nutritional values. Which is best?

The short answer is wholemeal, followed by brown, and then white. But what's the difference?

*Wholemeal bread* is made from the whole of the wheat grain, including the outer husk (bran), which is especially rich in fibre, and also the embryo wheat plant (wheatgerm) which is rich in nutrients. It has a natural brown colour and chewy texture. Its fibre content is 8.5 per cent.

*Brown bread* (sometimes called 'wheatmeal', a confusing term which is being phased out). The milling process has stripped away about half of the bran and wheatgerm, taking some fibre, protein and other nutrients with it. Vitamin B, iron and calcium have to be added to offset some of the losses. Caramel may be used to give the familiar brown colour, and other additives help to create a smoother texture and longer 'shelf life'. Its fibre content is 5.1 per cent.

*White bread* has lost most of its bran and wheatgerm in the flour mill. Nevertheless the white starchy grain remaining still contains useful amounts of fibre and protein. As with brown bread, vitamin B, iron and calcium must be added by law to replace those lost. Other additives provide the lighter, springier texture that so many consumers seem to want. Preservatives are added to improve the 'freshness' of the loaf. The fibre content is 2.7 per cent

Three other sorts of bread, 'wheatgerm', 'granary' and 'added bran' bread are worth mentioning here.

*Wheatgerm bread* is made from partially milled flour as for brown bread but has extra wheatgerm added. Fibre content 4.6 per cent.

*Granary bread* is made with a special flour blend containing partially-milled flour with malted wheat and rye flakes. Fibre content 5.2 per cent.

*Added bran bread* is white, brown or wheatgerm bread with extra bran added to increase the fibre content. Wheatgerm bread with added bran has the highest fibre level of all the widely available breads at 11.1 per cent.

● The second important point about bread is that it does contain rather a lot of salt. In fact, it's one of the main sources of salt in our diet (see page 25). Now, before you start agonising as to whether this cancels out all the good things about bread, let us hasten to say that you can eat plenty of bread and keep your salt intake down by being careful about the salt you add in cooking and at table, and choosing less salty foods in general. In other words, when you cut down your daily salt, spare your daily bread. Having said that, the bread manufacturers could do us all a favour by putting much less salt in bread. Perhaps in easy stages, starting from now.

● The third point is to make sure that you don't let your extra slices of bread mean lots of extra butter or margarine. Instead cut thicker and spread thinner. Better still, try your bread without any spread at all. You'll find that good quality wholemeal bread is just as tasty without it.

So our advice with Diet 2000 is to eat more bread, especially high-fibre bread such as wholemeal. Our Fill-up Formula on page 44 gives you a guide as to how much bread to eat. And on page 119 we tell you how you can make your own nutritious wholemeal loaves.

## Dairy foods

At the dairy counter, it's worth spending some time choosing very carefully indeed. After all, it's here that nearly half your intake of fat may be decided upon. Should it be butter or marge? And, if marge, which marge?

## Butter v. marge

This must be one of the longest running, and ugliest, battles on the food scene. The soft margarine people try to give the impression that their product is healthier than butter, particularly with regard to heart disease. The butter people say their product is natural, wholesome and harmless. They've both succeeded in one thing: confusing the public with a great greasy blob of conflicting information.

Which should it be?

*Point No.1* As far as calories are concerned, there's no significant difference between butter and margarine, whichever kind of margarine you're thinking of – soft or hard, sunflower or otherwise. BUT there are several low fat spreads in the shops that are not margarines in the strict sense of the word and DO have fewer calories than either butter or marge, because they contain a lot of water.

*Point No.2* By asking the question 'which should it be?' you're falling into the trap of thinking of particular foods as either 'good for you' or 'bad for you'. It may be easier to think of them that way but that's not how foods work when it comes to health. Of course, if you eat deadly nightshade berries they will poison you. But we're not talking about that kind of immediate effect; we mean the effect on your long-term health. What matters is the *overall* amount of such crucial components as saturated fat, salt, fibre and calorie count in your food over a period of time. Weeks and months as far as your weight is concerned. Years and decades for your general health and wellbeing. So ritual spreading of sunflower marge to stave off heart disease is no more than a mere token unless you make an effort to cut down on saturated fat right across the board, particularly in fatty meat, sausages, bacon, fried foods, milk and cheese.

*Point No.3* The less you spread on your bread, or use in cooking, the less reason there is for using a soft polyunsaturated margarine rather than butter or other margarines, because of the smaller part it plays in your overall fat consumption.

If you spread it thinly and use it sparingly or only occasionally, then it makes no real difference whether it's butter or marge. A *little* of what you fancy is good for the soul. But when it comes to your heart, a *lot* of what you fancy may do you harm.

*Point No.4* There are margarines . . . and margarines, when it comes to saturated fat content, as the table below shows.

Cooking fats and oils also differ greatly in their saturated fat content (see the table). Beware of cooking oils labelled 'blended vegetable oil'; these can be highly saturated.

## FATS AND OILS
- ● Saturated
- ○ Unsaturated

| | Total fat |
|---|---|
| Butter (salted) 10g spread on 1 slice bread | ●●●○ |
| Margarine hard, vegetable oils only (10g) | ●●○○ |
| soft, animal and vegetable oils only (10g) | ●●○○ |
| soft, vegetable oils only (10g) | ●●○○ |
| polyunsaturated (10g) | ●○○○ |
| Low fat spread 10g | ●○ |
| Oils 1 tablespoon coconut oil | ●●●●●●○ |
| cottonseed oil | ●●○○○○○ |
| maize (corn) oil | ●○○○○○○ |
| olive oil | ●○○○○○○ |
| palm oil | ●●●○○○○ |
| peanut oil | ●●○○○○○ |
| safflower seed oil | ●○○○○○○ |
| soya bean oil | ●○○○○○○ |
| sunflower seed oil | ●○○○○○ |

|  | Total fat |
|---|---|
| wheatgerm oil | ●○○○○○○○ |
| Dripping<br>½oz | ●●●○○○○○ |
| Lard<br>½oz | ●●●○○○○○ |
| Suet<br>shredded, 1oz | ●●●○○○○○ |

Still at the dairy counter . . .

## To skim or not to skim?

One-eighth of the fat the average Briton consumes comes from the daily ¾ pinta. So the question of whether to switch to skimmed or semi-skimmed is no mere fad, it's a way of making a big cut in fat without having to think too hard about it . . . all it takes is one note to the milkman. Here is a list of the different grades of milk with their fat content. To cut the fat you can either drink less milk, or switch to a lower fat grade, or do both.

Remember the fat in milk (called 'butterfat') is mostly saturated (63 per cent). With Diet 2000 you are aiming to halve your saturated fat intake, so a decision on milk could make quite a difference. And of course it will cut the calories too.

| Type of milk | Fat content |
|---|---|
| Gold top | 5% |
| Silver top | 4% |
| Semi-skimmed | 2% |
| Skimmed | Less than 1% |

More and more dairies are now delivering fresh skimmed and semi-skimmed milk to front doorsteps all over the country, as people become more fat-conscious. And all self-respecting supermarkets stock it too. Try it yourself, starting with the semi-skimmed. It's rather thinner than whole milk, but you'll find you soon get used to it.

## Cheese

For some strange reason, people think of cheese as a 'slimming'

53

food. Goodness know why, because cheeses contain a lot of fat. Look at this table of typical cheeses with their fat content . . . and go easy on a high fat cheese like Stilton or Cheddar.

| Type of cheese | Fat content |
| --- | --- |
| Cottage cheese | 4% |
| Cheese spread | 23% |
| Edam type | 23% |
| Camembert type | 23% |
| Processed cheese | 25% |
| Danish blue type | 29% |
| Cheddar type | 34% |
| Stilton type | 40% |
| Cream cheese | 47% |

## At the butcher

At the meat counter, select leaner cuts. True, they are more expensive but you can make up for that by buying less. Get the butcher to cut as much fat off as possible. Beware fatty mince, sausages, pies and pâtés. About half the fat in most meats and meat products is saturated. Choose chicken, turkey and perhaps rabbit as lower saturated fat alternatives. Or walk round the corner to the fishmongers. White fish have very little fat, and what there is in oily fish like herring and mackerel is mainly polyunsaturated.

## Wholefoods

If you're near a wholefood store, use it. You don't have to chant a mantra to get in. Ask for their unsweetened and unsalted muesli. Or better still, buy the ingredients and make it up yourself using our recipe on page 70. Experiment with pulses; there are dozens of different dried beans, peas and lentils that come to life after an overnight soak and are packed with protein and fibre. Try the wholewheat pasta and brown rice, and take home some wholemeal flour and bakers' yeast to make your own bread.

## Fruit and vegetables

It's well worth shopping around for produce in the best condition and best value for money. The longer fruit and vegetables are in storage, the more of their vitamin content they lose. Why not splash out on the occasional exotic fruit just for fun? There's nothing quite like mangoes on your muesli! Don't completely ignore frozen or canned fruit and vegetables. Sometimes they're just as nutritious, and maybe more so, than their 'fresh' alternatives. Frozen peas are a classic example. High in fibre, and, depending on the season, can contain more vitamin C than fresh peas. Canned fruit and vegetables can be high in fibre too but watch out for added sugar and salt. Generally speaking, fresh is best.

## In the kitchen: how to prepare and cook the most nutritious meals

This is where it all really happens for Diet 2000. Any amount of careful symbol counting and label reading and low fat, low sugar, low salt, high fibre food buying will come to nought if you don't get it right in the kitchen.

Our menus and recipes will give you plenty of ideas and guidance to keep you on the right tracks. But we thought it would be useful here to make a few general points about Diet 2000 cooking.

### Kitchen slave?

Don't get the idea that following Diet 2000 means you have to spend your life in the kitchen, grinding your way through sacks of grain, chopping cabbage upon cabbage and stirring endless fish stews. There's no reason why your cooking has to be more labour-intensive just because you're stepping away from lots of meat-based meals to more based on cereal, vegetables and fruit.

Here are a few labour-saving tips:

● *Make use of good convenience foods* This may surprise you after all we've said but many convenience foods are very nutritious. We've already mentioned frozen vegetables and how they can be high in fibre and vitamins. Frozen fish are also a useful and nutritious commodity. As a very rough and ready rule if you can recognise it when you get it out of the packet, then it's probably beneficial! If you can't, then it's probably a made-up meal and it's likely to be full of fat, salt or sugar and low in fibre.

- *Use your kitchen gear* For instance . . . If you've got a freezer, use it to the full. In quieter moments make up a plentiful supply of your favourite Diet 2000 dishes and store them away in the freezer for more frantic times. This also means that you can buy in bulk and save money. If you have a microwave cooker you can not only defrost fast, which can be a great boon, but can also bake potatoes in their jackets without destroying much vitamin C (which is mainly just under the skin). With a blender you can whizz up a whole range of wonderful mixtures: fruit drinks, vegetable purees like carrot, celery and cucumber, soups, dips and fillings. Needless to say a food processor does all that and more.

- *Keep a good store* To save you having to keep dashing to the shops as you prepare your Diet 2000 dishes, here are some additional items worth having in the larder or freezer:

| | |
|---|---|
| dried fruits | these are high fibre natural sweeteners and a whole range are easily available |
| dried pulses | lots of different sorts of beans, lentils and peas. They keep for ages in airtight jars |
| oatmeal | unsalted |
| nuts | use them fairly soon after purchase – they can go rancid |
| pasta: macaroni, spaghetti, lasagne | preferably wholewheat. Keeps for ages in airtight jars |
| rice | white and brown |
| bakers' yeast | |
| wholewheat crispbread | |
| fresh fruit, fresh vegetables | store in fridge |
| frozen fruit, vegetables and fish | these are good standbys and just as nutritious |
| tinned fruit | in natural juice |
| tinned vegetables | without added salt |
| tinned fish | e.g. tuna, sardines, pilchards |
| unsweetened fruit juices | without preservatives |

| | |
|---|---|
| dried skimmed milk | useful as a low fat alternative in some recipes and for tea/coffee. But fresh skimmed or semi-skimmed is better if you can get it |
| plain yogurt | it's low in fat |
| cottage cheese | and other low fat cheeses |
| corn oil<br>sunflower oil<br>safflower oil<br>soya oil<br>olive oil | all are relatively low in saturated fats |
| polyunsaturated margarine | in moderation |

## Healthy hints

Here are some simple hints for steering clear of fat, sugar and salt, and increasing the fibre in your diet.

**Fat**
- Choose fish and poultry which are low in fat more often than red meats
- Remove the skin from chicken and turkey
- Trim off visible fat and look for lean cuts when you do have red meat
- Use cooking foil to cook fish, poultry and meat in their own juices
- Skim off the fat from stews, casseroles and gravy
- Prepare dishes which combine meat with vegetables, cereals, pasta and pulses
- Serve smaller portions of meat
- Choose a cheese which is lower in fat, rather than Cheddar all the time
- Change over to semi-skimmed or skimmed milk
- Keep an eye on snack foods, they tend to be high in fat
- Grill rather than fry
- Try dry-frying in a non-stick pan
- If you must fry, use an oil low in saturated fat
- Use oil low in saturated fat for baking
- Beware baked goods which add a lot of fat to your diet, whether it's sweet items like biscuits or ready prepared meat pies

- Avoid rich, creamy sauces. Try natural low fat yogurt instead

## Fibre
- Whenever possible eat fruits in their skins and try to choose a fresh fruit as a dessert more often than not
- Use wholemeal flour in cooking
- Use wholemeal bread, wholegrain crispbreads
- Use wholegrain pasta and brown rice
- Choose a breakfast cereal that will give you plenty of fibre, without added sugar and salt
- Bake potatoes in their skins
- Eat more vegetables raw
- Cook vegetables very lightly, just enough to tenderise them

## Sugar
- Use fresh or dried fruits to sweeten desserts
- Cut down on sugar in baking

## Salt
- Avoid using stock cubes
- Salt does not need to be added automatically in cooking; leave it out and give the consumer a real choice
- Use lemon juice, herbs and spices to add flavour

### Get souped up
We've suggested lots of soups for Diet 2000. They're easy to make and can be done beforehand and kept in the larder or fridge. All you have to do is reheat them. Some can even be deep-frozen. Rather than use those little beef or chicken stock cubes (which are nearly all salt), we suggest you make your own stock, as a base for soups and many other dishes, by boiling bones, vegetables and vegetable peelings in a saucepan of water with a bouquet garni. Then cool the stock and remove the fat before you add other ingredients. And go easy on the salt!

### Sandwich fillings
When choosing sandwich fillings go for the low-fat choices: thinly sliced chicken or fish, a lower fat cheese or fat-free cheese. Increase the quantities of salad items used in sandwich combinations. Cut the cucumber thicker and spread the salmon thinner in the Sunday tea sandwiches. Or be more generous with the tomato than the cheese

when making up rolls with that combination.

**Open faced sandwiches**

These usually comprise a selection of fillings displayed to be particularly attractive: a thin slice of smoked salmon with a lemon twist on rye crispbread; or cottage cheese with pineapple on wholemeal; asparagus tips, attractively garnished; the possibilities are infinitely appetising.

## *Quick guide to herbs and spices*

*Herbs*

| | |
|---|---|
| Basil | vegetable soups; tomato soup; beef stew; fish; on fresh sliced tomatoes; on stewed tomatoes, aubergine, asparagus, broccoli; on bread |
| Bay leaves | soups and stews |
| Caraway | pork; coleslaw; cabbage, turnips; rye and pumpernickel bread |
| Chives | with cabbage, potatoes, courgettes; omelettes |
| Dill | as garnish on fish; potato salad; sliced cucumber; with beans, cabbage, cauliflower, potatoes |
| Fennel | with fish; sliced tomato, onion; in bread |
| Garlic | salads; savoury dishes |
| Marjoram | soups; stews; grilled or baked fish; with chicken, veal, lamb; in scones |
| Mint | with lamb; in pea soup; in salads; in fruit drinks |
| Oregano | in tomato juice or soups; meat sauces; meat balls; pizzas |
| Parsley | as garnish on savouries; meats; fish |
| Rosemary | in chicken, spinach or pea soup; on chicken, lamb or veal; in baked fish; in salad dressings; potato salad |
| Sage | in consommé or cream soups; on poultry or pork; with beans |
| Tarragon | in salad dressings, sauces; with fish, chicken, savouries |
| Thyme | in soups; with fish; in dumplings |

*Spices*

| | |
|---|---|
| Allspice | with tomato and pea soups; in roasts or marinades; in poached fish; on fruit salad; in salad dressings |

| Cinnamon | on lamb chops; in stews; on tomatoes; on cottage cheese; over oranges, bananas, berries and apples |
| Cloves | in borscht, split pea, potato soup; baked fish; on beans, cucumber, tomatoes; in apple and pear desserts |
| Ginger | on chicken dishes; on pears; on beetroots, carrots, cucumber; in fruit salad |
| Mace | in casseroles, in sauces for vegetables |
| Mustard | in casseroles, meat loaves, hamburgers, sausages or roast beef |
| Nutmeg | with chicken soup; in meat loaf; on chicken; in fishcakes; on carrots, beans, spinach, peas; in fruit salad; on custard |
| Paprika | as garnish in soups and on raw vegetables; on chicken and veal; on fish; on creamed vegetables |

## *Diet 2000 tips for chips*

Cut thicker chips. The thinner they are, the bigger the surface area and the more fat they absorb.

Avoid crinkle-cut chips. Again, there is more surface area fat to soak into.

Choose the right oil. It must be a low saturated fat oil (sometimes labelled 'high in polyunsaturates') such as corn oil, sunflower oil, safflower oil.

Cook them hot. Use a trial chip or two to test the temperature. Chips should really sizzle rather than soak up the fat.

Drain well. Tap the scoop to shed excess fat.

Serve on paper. Not newspaper à la fish and chip shop, but a double layer of kitchen roll to blot away the last remaining blobs.

Then turn on to the plate. What would life be without chips!

Here's what a difference you can make:

A portion of typical chips cooked in lard

fat content ○○○○○●●●●

A portion of Diet 2000 chips

fat content ○○○●

And remember to use vinegar or lemon juice rather than salt.


## Cooking with pulses

Using pulses, peas, beans and lentils, had come to be looked on as rather old fashioned or just plain odd, at one stage. But now once again they have come into their own as a terrific source of fibre, as well as protein and other nutrients, which are available all year round. So some of us have to relearn the rules about cooking these foods, things our mothers perhaps would not have had to think twice about.

Dried pulses (except lentils and split peas) need pre-soaking. Either i) bring them to the boil in a large pan of *un*salted water, boil for three to five minutes, turn off heat and leave to soak for at least an hour or ii) soak them in three times their volume of cold water for four to six hours or overnight.

If beans tend to give you wind, it may help to discard the soaking water and cook in fresh water, though you will be discarding some vitamins as well.

The cooking time for pulses varies quite widely and a rough guide is given overleaf.

Most of that cooking time will be at a steady simmer, but for the red kidney beans particularly it is important that they are actually boiling for at least ten minutes of the cooking time in order to destroy the naturally occurring toxins.

For just the right dietary combination, team pulses with grains, wholemeal flour and bread. It seems that beans on toast has a lot going for it –more than perhaps you realised.

| Type | Approximate cooking time of soaked beans |
|---|---|
| Adzuki | 30 minutes |
| Black beans | 1 hour |
| Black-eyed beans | 30–45 minutes |
| Borlotti beans | 1 hour |
| Broad beans | 1½ hours |
| Butter beans | 1¼ hours |
| Cannelini beans | 1 hour |
| Chick peas | 1–1½ hours |
| Flageolet beans | 1 hour |
| Haricot beans | 1–1½ hours |
| Lima beans | 45–60 minutes |
| Mung beans | 20–30 minutes |
| Pinto beans | 1–1¼ hours |
| Red kidney beans | 1 hour |
| Soya beans | 3–4 hours |

# The Diet 2000 menus

The sample weeks' menus aim to show you how foods can be combined to meet the NACNE targets. How much of the accompaniments you should be eating – bread, vegetables, fruit, etc., can be calculated using the Fill-Up Formula on page 44.

You will see that many of the dishes suggested have an asterisk, which means that a recipe has been provided. By using these recipes you can enjoy a wide variety of foods and still meet the NACNE targets.

If you were to substitute a commercially prepared version of one of the dishes (nip into the pub for a shepherd's pie, for example, instead of making it from the recipe), you should make allowances somewhere else in that day's or week's intake for the extra fat and salt it contains.

But these are only suggestions, not hard and fast rules. They may give you ideas for new recipes, or for modifying your old favourites.

Here are some more ideas you might like to try out to make your own recipes more nutritious:

1 Replace whole milk with skimmed milk.
2 When making cakes, convert your own solid fat recipes – you'll find you need between a quarter and a third less corn oil than butter or margarine.
3 Using wholemeal varieties is an easy way to improve spaghetti and macaroni dishes.
4 When baking or making pastry, try replacing the flour with wholemeal flour.
5 Or try making pastry without fat, as suggested in the recipe on page 88.
6 Look at the amount of sugar a recipe calls for – you could probably halve that without complaints from the family.
7 What about the salt the recipe suggests adding? Why not leave it out and let the consumers decide for themselves? They may not notice at all; and if the 'added salt habit' is a reflex action in your family at least you will have halved the amount of salt they are eating.

8  Look at the amount of meat you usually use in a favourite recipe.
   What about replacing some of that by adding extra vegetables?
   Not only will it make the dish healthier, but the pennies will go
   further as well.
9  What about the cheese you choose to cook with? Could you use a
   lower fat variety or perhaps add a little dry mustard? It will
   enhance the flavour and make a small quantity of cheese go
   further.
10 Plain yogourt can be used in many recipes in place of cream or
   sour cream to reduce the fat content.

## Spring menu

Spring brings a range of fresh fruit and vegetables at their best to our
tables: new potatoes, broccoli and rhubarb are just some that feature
in the menu for this season. Perhaps it's also worth thinking about
growing some vegetables of your own; this could give you unusual
vegetables at a reasonable cost, as well as an enjoyable leisure
activity.

Some days feel like summer and some like the darkest days of
winter at this time of year and suggestions have been included which
should suit the season; whatever the weather is doing outside, this
sort of food will be doing you good inside.

## Summer menu

Now is the time to go to town with fresh fruit, without breaking the
bank. What a delicious variety to choose from: strawberries, raspberries, gooseberries, plums, peaches and apricots. Delicious on
their own, or perhaps made up into one of the special desserts
featured in this season's menu as a treat.

Summer also means a chance to eat outside with barbecues and
picnics. Our suggestion for Sunday lunch can easily be packed up
and taken to a pleasant spot on a sunny day. While on Saturday you
may enjoy a barbecue with friends – and even if you don't have the
equipment to cook out of doors, these delicious kebabs can easily be
made on a traditional cooker and served outside in the sunshine.

## Autumn menu

There's a whole harvest of fruit and vegetables available at this time of year, a chance to try some new combinations with a favourite dish or try a new recipe that makes a satisfying meal based on vegetables. If you want to make the most of this season of plenty, the effort of bottling or freezing now could pay dividends later, by adding variety to your winter choice at a reasonable price.

With the evenings drawing in and a nip in the air, appetites sharpen for warming soups and more filling fare. Here are some suggestions for enjoyable meals that won't load you down with fat, sugar and salt at the same time.

## Winter menu

Convenience foods are not necessarily a bad thing. After all, there's nothing more convenient than a frozen pea and freezing has made available to us a whole host of foods on a year-round basis that can help us to eat in a healthier way. The ingredients preserved by the older process of drying also come into their own at this time of year when peas, beans and lentils can turn a simple soup into a satisfying meal, as some of the suggested recipes show.

Food is always a great comforter, especially on gloomy winter days; the sort of meals we've suggested aim to cheer you through the cold and wet with the added bonus that you won't have to go on a crash diet next spring to get rid of the extra weight you've put on.

| Sunday | Monday | Tuesday | Wednesday | Thursday | Friday | Saturday |
|---|---|---|---|---|---|---|
| Apple cinnamon pancakes* | Bran & raisin muffins | Muesli supreme* | Porridge* | Cereal cocktail* | Muesli* | ½ grapefruit<br>Poached egg on wholemeal toast<br>Grilled bacon<br>Grilled tomato |
| Fruit juice | Dried fruit compôte* | Wholemeal toast | Wholemeal toast | Wholemeal toast | Wholemeal toast | |
| Roast lamb<br>Saucy leeks*<br>Spring greens<br>New potatoes | Spring vegetable soup* | Cream of asparagus soup* | Lentil soup* | Macaroni cheese | Red bean soup* | Pea soup* |
| | Granary rolls with cheese & tomato<br>Waldorf salad | Cornish pasty*<br>Coleslaw | Tuna salad sandwiches on wholemeal bread | Tomato salad<br>Sweetcorn niblets | Chicken sandwiches on wholemeal bread<br>Potato salad | Stuffed jacket potato*<br>Green salad |
| Rhubarb crunch*<br>Orange sauce* | Fresh fruit | Fresh fruit | Fresh fruit | Fresh fruit | Fresh fruit | Fresh fruit |
| Salmon & cucumber sandwiches | Stuffed cabbage leaves*<br>Brown rice | Liver casserole*<br>Carrots<br>Mashed potatoes<br>Peas | Spaghetti bolognese* | Chicken paprika<br>Broccoli<br>Mashed potatoes | Chinese baked fish*<br>Brown rice<br>Beansprout salad | Pizza* |
| Fruit salad<br>Fresh fruit cake | Sweetcorn<br>Banana surprise* | Rhubarb & orange mousse* | Apple cobbler* | Citrus circles* | Tropical fruit salad* | Baked apple |

## SUMMER SUGGESTIONS

| Sunday | Monday | Tuesday | Wednesday | Thursday | Friday | Saturday |
|---|---|---|---|---|---|---|
| Two fruit whizz* | Muesli with strawberries* | Wheat crunch* | Melon and grape cocktail | Wholewheat cereal with sliced banana | Sliced fresh peaches with granola* | Wholewheat cereal |
| Oatmeal and raisin fingers* | Wholemeal toast | Wholemeal toast | Sunrise muffins* | Wholemeal toast | Wholemeal toast | Scrambled eggs on wholemeal toast |
| Gazpacho* Cold chicken Potato salad Mixed summer salad Wholemeal rolls | Pineapple and cottage cheese platter Granary roll | Meat loaf (cold)* Tasty tomatoes Baked potatoes Cauliflower salad | Chicken sandwiches on wholemeal bread | Summer soup* Tomato sandwiches on wholemeal bread | Bean and cottage cheese flan* Green salad Wholemeal roll | Kebabs* Wholemeal pitta bread Green salad |
| Summer pudding | Fresh fruit | Individual raspberry crisp | Fresh fruit | Fresh fruit | Fresh fruit | Fresh fruit |
| Egg and tomato sandwiches | Savoury filled pancakes* | Asparagus flan* Tomato salad | Stuffed green peppers* Brown rice | Quick kedgeree* Cucumber relish Wholemeal chapattis | Deep dish chicken and corn pie* Mange tout peas Mashed potatoes | Cheese and cucumber sandwiches |
| Strawberry sponge cake* | Gooseberry fool* | Fresh fruit | Peach Melba pie* | Fresh fruit salad | Apricot raspberry yogurt* | Raspberry cups |

## AUTUMN SUGGESTIONS

| | Sunday | Monday | Tuesday | Wednesday | Thursday | Friday | Saturday |
|---|---|---|---|---|---|---|---|
| | Dried fruit compôte* <br> Wholegrain cereal <br> Wholemeal toast | Apple oatmeal* <br> Wholemeal toast | Muesli* <br> Wholemeal toast | Porridge* <br> Boiled egg <br> Wholemeal toast | Wholewheat cereal with sliced banana <br> Wholemeal toast | Blackberry granola* <br> Wholemeal toast | ½ grapefruit <br> Hot scones with thick fruit purée |
| | Roast chicken <br> Rice stuffing* <br> Cauliflower <br> Ratatouille* <br> Mashed potatoes <br> Blackberry and apple pie* <br> Custard* | Chicken noodle soup* <br> Three bean salad <br> Wholemeal roll <br> Fresh fruit | Fisherman's pie* <br> Runner beans <br> Sweetcorn <br> Plum crunch | Bean soup* <br> Autumn salad plate <br> Wholemeal roll | Lasagne* <br> Zucchini toss <br> Fresh fruit salad | Fresh tomato soup* <br> Onion tart* <br> Beansprout and orange salad <br> Granary roll | Chilli con carne <br> Brown rice <br> Corn on the cob <br> Green salad <br> Wholemeal garlic bread <br> Stewed blackcurrants <br> Custard* |
| | Open faced sandwiches <br> Spicy apple cake* | Quick chicken curry <br> Chapattis <br> Brown rice <br> Dhal <br> Autumn fruit salad | Broccoli casserole* <br> Sweetcorn salad <br> Fresh fruit | Baked stuffed marrow* <br> Brown rice <br> Apple snow | Scottish fish soup* <br> Oatcakes <br> Fresh fruit | Italian veal casserole* <br> Wholewheat noodles <br> Green salad <br> Baked pears | Savoury scones <br> Celery stalks <br> Tomato salad |

## WINTER SUGGESTIONS

| Sunday | Monday | Tuesday | Wednesday | Thursday | Friday | Saturday |
|---|---|---|---|---|---|---|
| Cereal with fruit<br>Baked beans on wholemeal toast | Wholewheat cereal with fruit<br>Wholemeal toast | Muesli*<br>Wholemeal toast | Porridge*<br>Wholemeal toast | Cereal cocktail*<br>Wholemeal toast | Wholewheat cereal with fruit<br>Wholemeal toast | Potato cakes*<br>Grilled tomatoes<br>Grilled bacon |
| Roast beef Yorkshire pudding<br>Crunchy parsnips*<br>Mashed potatoes<br>French beans | Leek and potato soup*<br>Wholemeal salad roll | Tuna-noodle casserole*<br>Celery and green pepper salad | Curried lentil soup*<br>Granary roll with herring roe pâté* | Savoury leek pie*<br>Baked beans | Split pea soup*<br>Cheese and tomato granary roll | Chicken casserole*<br>Brown rice<br>Carrots |
| Satsuma delight* | Fresh fruit | Apricot and orange mousse* | Fresh fruit | Spiced pears | Apple cinnamon yoghurt* | Stewed plums and custard |
| Open-faced sandwiches<br>Peas<br>Carrots | Shepherd's pie*<br>Peas<br>Carrots | Winter warmer soup*<br>Savoury toasts | Spanish omelette*<br>Green salad | Minestrone soup* | Fish and chips<br>Peas | Sardine fingers |
| Banana and raisin teabread* | Apple charlotte* | Fruit | Spicy bread pudding* with orange sauce* | Sausage roll*<br>Pasta crunch* | Winter fruit salad | Honey bread* with apricot relish* |

# The Diet 2000 recipes

*Note*:
All recipes are based on serving four people except in the case of cakes and bulk productions like granola and muesli.

All scoring is per portion.

Ingredients are given in metric and imperial measurements. Use one system or the other, but do not mix the two in one recipe, as the quantities are not interchangeable.

## Breakfasts

*Cereal cocktail*

Some commercial breakfast cereals are high in fibre and low in salt and sugar. Why not ring the changes by mixing some of these together? Add in extra dried fruit, fresh fruit or nuts as the fancy takes you.

## Muesli

Commercial muesli often has a lot of added sucrose, which is why it is a good thing to choose your breakfast cereal carefully or make your own muesli. It can easily be made up in bulk for convenience and you can make your own variations by adding dried apple flakes, etc. It can be served in a variety of ways, with fresh fruit or fruit juice instead of the more traditional milk, or with plain yogurt.

225 g/8 oz rolled oat flakes
225 g/8 oz rolled wheat flakes
225 g/8 oz rolled barley flakes
100 g/4 oz wheatgerm
160 g/6 oz mixed chopped nuts
160 g/6 oz sultanas or raisins

Mix the flakes and wheatgerm together, then add the nuts and dried fruit. Store in an airtight jar.

# Muesli supreme

♦ ♦ ♦ ♦                🝙🝙🝙🝙                                   🌾🌾🌾🌾

This mixture will set you up for the day, giving you plenty of energy and fibre.

2 × 150 g/5 oz cartons natural
   yogurt
50 g/2 oz raisins
50 g/2 oz chopped nuts

225 g/8 oz oatmeal
2 tbsp orange juice
1 medium apple, sliced
2 medium bananas, sliced

Mix all ingredients. Vary fruits according to availability.

# Apple oatmeal

♦                 🝙                                       🌾🌾

This Mennonite recipe gives a new slant to a very familiar breakfast food and helps to increase the fibre content.

100 g/4 oz rolled oats
½ tsp salt
225 ml/8 fl oz water

2 medium apples, peeled and
   chopped
Dash nutmeg

Combine the oats, salt and water in a saucepan and cook for 10 minutes on a low heat. Add the apples and nutmeg and cook for 5 minutes more, or until apples are done to desired consistency. Serve with skimmed milk or yogurt.

# Wheat crunch

🝙             🌾

Wheat crunch has a similar texture to grapenuts and can be used in many of the same ways: as a breakfast cereal on its own, combined with fruit or as a topping on a crunchy fruit pudding.

| 400 g/14 oz wholemeal flour | 455 ml/16 fl oz buttermilk or |
| 85 g/3 oz wheatgerm | plain yogurt |
| 50 g/2 oz brown sugar | |

Combine all the ingredients in a large mixing bowl. Beat until smooth. Spread dough on two large greased baking sheets. Bake at 180°C/350°F/Gas Mark 4 for 25–30 minutes. Crumble by one of the following methods:

i) While still warm, break into chunks and grate or whirl briefly in the blender, about a cupful at a time.

ii) Allow to cool thoroughly, then put through a food grinder using a coarse plate.

Crisp in the oven at 120°C/250°F/Gas Mark ½ for about 20 minutes. Cool and store in an airtight container. Eat with milk or stewed fruit.

# Porridge

Porridge is traditionally made with added salt but you may find that you still enjoy it made with much less than the usual amount, or none at all. There are plenty of ways of serving porridge as well, apart from with the conventional salt or sugar and milk. Try sprinkling some mixed dried fruit on the top, to add sweetness, but in its natural form – wrapped in fibre.

1 litre/1¾ pints water
100 g/4 oz rolled oats
1 tsp salt

Measure the water into a pan. Add the oats and salt and stir while bringing to the boil. Simmer for 4 minutes, stirring occasionally.

# Potato cakes

There's no reason why you can't have something fried occasionally and these potato cakes team up nicely with grilled bacon and tomato for a change.

900 g/2 lb potatoes
1 egg
50 g/2 oz chopped onions

3 tbsp wholemeal flour
25 g/1 oz margarine

Wash the potatoes, peel, and remove eyes. Shred the potatoes and drain thoroughly. Beat the egg until thick and lemon coloured. Mix in the potatoes, onion and flour. Melt the margarine in a frying pan over low heat. Shape the potato mixture into 8 cakes and place in the pan. Cook over medium heat, turning once, until golden brown and cooked through, about 5 minutes.

# Granola

800 g/1¾ lb rolled oats
50 g/2 oz chopped nuts
100 g/4 oz raisins
50 g/2 oz wheatgerm

50 g/2 oz powdered skimmed
  milk
2 tbsp honey
2 tbsp corn oil
1 tsp vanilla essence

Preheat oven to 180°C/350°F/Gas Mark 4. Place the oats in an ungreased 22.5×32.5 cm/9×13 inch pan and bake for 10 minutes. Remove from the oven and stir in the nuts, raisins, wheatgerm and powdered skimmed milk. Add the honey, corn oil and vanilla essence and stir until thoroughly coated. Bake for 10–15 minutes, stirring every 3 minutes or so, until uniformly golden. Do not overbake. Let cool in the pan undisturbed, then break into chunks. Store in an airtight container.

# Oatmeal and raisin fingers

Use basic recipe for granola and add:
1 beaten egg
50 ml/2 fl oz skimmed milk

Stir the liquid ingredients into the dry ones and mix well. Press the mixture firmly into two well greased 25×37.5 cm/10×15 inch baking trays. Bake at 180°C/350°F/Gas Mark 4 until nicely browned. Cut immediately into fingers. Remove from the pans when cool.

# Hot scones

These scones are delicious served fresh from the oven with mashed banana or apple purée. A really healthy way to start the day.

225 g/8 oz wholemeal flour
4 tsp baking powder
½ tsp salt
½ tsp mixed spice

40 g/1½ oz margarine
25 g/1 oz sultanas
1 apple, peeled and grated
75 ml/2½ fl oz skimmed milk

Set the oven to 230°C/450°F/Gas Mark 8. Mix the flour, baking powder, salt and mixed spice. Rub in the margarine. Add the sultanas and grated apple. Mix well, then add the milk and mix to make a soft dough. Roll out on a floured board to 2 cm/¾ inch thick. Cut into rounds with a scone cutter and place on a baking tray. Brush with a little skimmed milk. Bake on the second shelf for about 10 minutes.

# Sunrise muffins

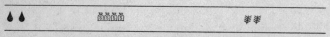

Orange juice, or other fruit juice, adds natural sweetness to these muffins and an interesting flavour.

| | |
|---|---|
| 250 g/9 oz wholemeal flour | 1 egg, beaten |
| 2 tsp baking powder | 50 ml/2 fl oz corn oil |
| ½ tsp salt | 340 ml/12 fl oz orange juice |

Combine the dry ingredients. Combine the wet ingredients. Fold wet and dry together quickly, just until the flour is moistened. Spoon into greased muffin tins. Bake at 200°C/400°F/Gas Mark 6 for about 20 minutes.

# Apple cinnamon pancakes

Pancakes are a nice way to start the day and can make a valuable contribution to your fibre intake as well if you use wholemeal flour instead of white. The tasty filling suggested also provides some fibre and is a healthier alternative to syrups or sugar. By using skimmed instead of full fat milk you can keep the fat content lower, without changing the taste.

| | |
|---|---|
| 100 g/4 oz wholemeal flour | *Filling* |
| Pinch salt | 3 large cooking apples |
| 1 egg | ½ tsp ground cinnamon |
| 250 ml/½ pint skimmed milk | 75 g/3 oz raisins |

To make pancakes, mix the flour and salt together and make a well in the centre. Break in the egg, add half the milk and beat well. When the batter is smooth, stir in the remainder of the milk. Beat well and leave to stand for at least 30 minutes.

To make the filling, coarsely grate the apple skins to remove. Core and slice the apples. Place the grated skin and fruit in a small saucepan and stew until softened, then add cinnamon and raisins. Mix thoroughly.

To cook the pancakes, heat a heavy-based non-stick pan, until a water droplet skitters across the surface before evaporating. Pour a little of the batter into the pan and tilt so that the mixture covers the base. Cook until the pancake starts to bubble, turn over and cook on the other side. Keep the pancakes warm until all have been prepared. Divide the warm filling between the pancakes, roll them up and serve.

# Two fruit whizz

A really refreshing way to start the day with all the natural fibre of these two citrus fruits.

3 oranges
2 grapefruits

Peel the fruit; don't worry too much about the amount of pith clinging to the fruit. Chop the flesh roughly and place in the blender. Whizz to a smooth consistency. This tastes even better if set aside in the fridge for a while to chill.

# Dried fruit compôte

This just goes to show you don't have to add spoonfuls of sugar to enjoy sweetness. Natural sweetness comes wrapped up in fibre to even up the score.

300 g/10 oz mixed dried fruit
Grated rind and juice of 1 lemon
200 ml/7 fl oz unsweetened
    orange juice

Soak the fruit in water overnight. Measure out 300 ml/½ pint of the soaking water into a saucepan; add the lemon rind and juice, orange juice and fruit. Bring slowly to the boil, cover and simmer for 30 minutes. This compôte can be served either hot or chilled.

# Soups

## Chicken stock

Chicken and vegetable stock can be made in larger batches and frozen (in ice trays if liked) for extra convenience.

| | |
|---|---|
| Chicken carcass | A few stalks parsley |
| 1 onion | 1 bay leaf |
| 2 carrots, sliced | 6 black peppercorns |
| 4 stalks celery, sliced | |

Put the chicken bones in a large saucepan, pour on 2.25/4 pints of water, cover and bring slowly to the boil. Skim off the scum that rises to the surface. Add the vegetables, bay leaf and peppercorns. Cover and return to the boil. Simmer for about 3 hours by which time the liquid will probably be reduced by half. Strain and allow the liquid to cool. Discard the remains of bones and vegetables. When cool, skim off the layer of fat on the surface.

## Vegetable stock

| | |
|---|---|
| 2 large onions | 1 large leek |
| 2 large carrots | 1 bouquet garni |
| 4 sticks celery | 6 black peppercorns |
| 1 small turnip | |

Clean and slice the vegetables. Add to about 2.25/4 pints of water in a large saucepan and cover. Bring to the boil. Skim off the scum as it rises. Add the bouquet garni and peppercorns, cover and return to the boil. Simmer for about 3 hours, or until the liquid is reduced by half. Strain and discard remains.

# Chicken noodle soup

◊      ❧

Chicken noodle soup is one of the most popular packet mix soups, and yet it could not be simpler to make fresh – and avoid all that salt.

900 ml/1½ pints chicken stock
  (see page 77)
50 g/2 oz vermicelli
1 tbsp chopped parsley

Bring the stock to the boil. Crumble in the vermicelli. Add chopped parsley, cook for about 5 minutes and serve.


# Cream of asparagus soup

◊      ❧

Asparagus sounds rather extravagant, but it is one of the vegetables that you might like to try growing yourself. Making creamy soups without a lot of butter or cream by using skimmed milk as suggested can be applied to other vegetables as well. This approach keeps the fat content down while keeping the flavour right.

| | |
|---|---|
| 1 bundle fresh asparagus or 1<br>    large (500 g/16 oz) tin<br>    asparagus | 2 tbsp cornflour<br>Pepper<br>Chopped parsley to garnish |
| 1 small onion | |
| 900 ml/1½ pints skimmed milk | *Option* |
| 3 tbsp cold skimmed milk | 1 tbsp plain yogurt |

Cut the asparagus into small pieces and chop the onion. Simmer the vegetables in the milk until they are tender, about 30 minutes. Mix the cornflour and cold milk to a smooth paste. Place the vegetable mixture in the blender and mix until smooth in consistency. Return to the saucepan. Add the cornflour paste and bring back to the boil, stirring continuously, season and simmer for 2 minutes. Serve garnished with chopped parsley.

*Option*: before serving, swirl in plain yogurt and garnish with chopped parsley.

# Lentil soup

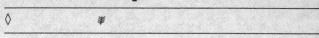

Lentil soup is filling, low in fat and a useful source of fibre.

| | |
|---|---|
| 1 large carrot | 1.5 litres/2½ pints water or |
| 1 large potato | stock |
| 1 medium onion | 75 g/3 oz dried skimmed milk |
| 160 g/6 oz brown lentils | Pepper |

Wash the vegetables and removed the onion skin. Dice the onion, potato and carrot and put them with the lentils and water or stock in a thick-bottomed saucepan. Bring to the boil slowly and simmer gently for about 2 hours. Mix all the ingredients (including the dried milk) in the blender until the soup is the desired consistency. Return to the pan, season with freshly milled pepper and serve piping hot.

# Scottish fish soup

This satisfying soup is almost a meal in itself.

| | |
|---|---|
| 1 onion | 450 g/1 lb mashed potato |
| 225 g/8 oz fresh haddock | Pepper |
| 600 ml/1 pint skimmed milk | |

Chop the onion finely. Place the haddock and the onion in a pan with just enough water to cover. Cook gently for about 10 minutes until the fish is beginning to flake away from the bones. Remove the fish, flake the flesh and put the bones back in the pan to cook gently for about an hour. Remove bones. Add the fish and milk to the fish stock. Add the mashed potato and stir to a thick creamy consistency. Season and serve.

# Red bean soup

❦❦❦❦

A soup which can be made very quickly and is a satisfying source of fibre and protein.

900 ml/1½ pints vegetable stock (see page 77)
1 large potato
1 medium onion
50 g/2 oz cooked (or tinned) red kidney beans

Black pepper
Lemon juice
Chopped parsley

Place the stock in a saucepan (or pressure cooker for a faster soup). Peel and roughly chop the potato and onion and add to the pan. Wash the red beans if tinned and add, stirring to distribute the beans. Cook until the vegetables are tender (about 10 minutes if using a pressure cooker). Cool, liquidise and return to the cooker. Reheat and season with pepper and lemon juice. Garnish with parsley.

# Curried lentil soup

Basic ❦
+ ◊ if option chosen

The basic soup is easy to make and provides fibre while being low in salt and fat. The optional extras will make it deliciously different but will also increase the fat content.

| 160 g/6 oz red or yellow lentils | *Option* |
| 900 ml/1½ pints of water | 1 medium onion |
| ½ tsp curry powder | 1 tsp freshly grated ginger |
| ½ tsp turmeric | 1 tbsp vegetable oil |
| 2 bay leaves | Garam masala |

Pick over the lentils to remove any small stones or other debris and wash well. Place in a strong saucepan with the water, curry powder, turmeric and bay leaves. Bring to the boil. Turn heat down and simmer gently, covered, for about 45 minutes or until the lentils are soft. Liquidise and add water to adjust consistency. Reheat and serve.

*Option*: peel and slice the onion and fry with the grated ginger in the oil until golden brown. Mix into the soup and sprinkle garam masala on the top before serving.

# Pea soup

🌢🌢                    ◊                    🌾🌾🌾🌾🌾

This filling soup contains a lot of fat in relation to its fibre content but will have a much lower salt content than commercially produced pea soups.

| 160 g/6 oz dried peas | 1 tbsp corn oil |
| 1.2 litres/2 pints water | Pepper |
| 1 large onion | Bouquet garni |
| 1 small carrot | 140 ml/¼ pint skimmed milk |
| ½ turnip | |

Wash the peas and soak overnight in the water. Peel and chop the other vegetables, lightly fry them in the oil for about 5 minutes. Add the soaked peas, the water in which they were soaked, the seasoning and bouquet garni. Cover and allow to simmer gently for 1½ to 2 hours. Remove the bouquet garni, stir in the milk, reheat and serve. (For a smoother soup you may prefer to blend it in the liquidiser, before adding the milk.)

# Spring vegetable soup

Ⓢ        ❀

Making stock yourself means that the salt content will be lower than in commercial stock cubes and any fat can be skimmed off when the stock cools. Adding pearl barley to soups helps to make them more satisfying and increases the fibre content.

850 ml/1½ pints chicken stock
  (see page 77)
25 g/1 oz pearl barley (soaked
  overnight and drained)
1 small carrot

1 small onion
1 stick celery
½ small turnip
Chopped parsley

Put the stock and barley together in a pan, bring to the boil and allow to simmer until cereal is cooked, about 1 hour. Meanwhile prepare the other vegetables, cutting them into cubes. When the cereal is cooked, add the vegetables and simmer until the vegetables are tender (about 10 minutes). Garnish with parsley.

# Gazpacho

⬤ ⬤ ⬤       ❀❀

Gazpacho is a cool refreshing soup for summer and makes use of plentiful salad vegetables in a rather different way.

450 g/1 lb tomatoes
1 clove garlic
1 green pepper
½ cucumber, peeled
2–3 tbsp lemon juice

Cayenne pepper
3 tbsp corn oil
Slices of lemon to garnish
  (optional)

Chop all the vegetables and mix in the blender. Add the lemon juice, cayenne pepper and oil, a little at a time, tasting to check that the soup is not too oily. Chill well in the refrigerator and serve garnished with lemon slices.

# Summer soup

This light and summery soup can be delicious on the 'not so warm'
days of an English summer; it's economical and will give some fibre.

½ large cucumber
225 g/8 oz spring onions
½ bunch watercress
1 tbsp corn oil

1.5 litres/2½ pints vegetable
  stock (see page 77)
25 g/1 oz wholemeal flour
1 tbsp skimmed milk
Chopped parsley

Slice the cucumber very finely, skin included. Shred the spring
onions and watercress, taking care to remove tough stems. Heat the
oil gently in a saucepan (not too hot), mix in the vegetables and
warm on a very low flame or a hot plate which has been heated but is
now turned off. Gentle heat like this, for about 15 minutes, brings
out the full flavour. Add the stock, bring to the boil and simmer for
an hour. Mix the flour into a thin paste with the milk, add to the
soup and boil for 5 minutes. Top with finely chopped parsley to
serve.


# Bean soup

A satisfying soup that is simple to make and nutritious.

225 g/8 oz navy beans
1.2 litres/2 pints water
1 onion, chopped
3 stalks celery, chopped

1 carrot, sliced
450 g/1 lb stewed tomatoes
Pepper

Soak the beans in the water overnight. Add the other vegetables and
simmer until the beans are tender, about 2 hours (can be speeded up
by using a pressure cooker). Season with pepper to taste.

# Fresh tomato soup

❀

When you have tasted real tomato soup you may wonder why you ever bothered with the 'convenient' variety – it will be better for you as well.

| | |
|---|---|
| 225 g/8 oz tomatoes | Pepper |
| 1 onion | 1 tbsp tomato purée (if needed) |
| 1 clove garlic | 1 tbsp skimmed milk |
| 600 ml/1 pint stock (see page 77) | Chives or spring onion tops |
| Bay leaf | |

Chop the tomatoes roughly, without removing their skins. Chop the onion and garlic quite finely. Bring the stock to the boil and add the vegetables and bay leaf. Simmer, covered, until the onion is soft. Remove bay leaf, put in blender and mix. Return to pan and simmer for 1 minute. Taste and add pepper and tomato purée, if needed. Stir in a little skimmed milk before serving. Garnish with a few chopped chives or spring onion tops.


# Leek and potato soup

❀❀❀

This soup makes good use of winter vegetables to provide the basis for a meal that's right on target for fat, fibre and salt.

| | |
|---|---|
| 3 large leeks, trimmed and chopped | 900 ml/1½ pints vegetable stock (see page 77) |
| 450 g/1 lb potatoes, chopped | Black pepper |
| 1 small onion, sliced | |

Simmer the leeks, potatoes and onion in the stock, in a covered pan, until tender, about 15-20 minutes. Place in the blender and mix. Return to the pan, season and reheat.

# Winter warmer soup

◊                 🌿🌿

Pearl barley is a traditional addition to soups which gives them more 'body'; it helps to add more fibre too.

75 g/3 oz pearl barley, soaked
   overnight and drained
1.2 litres/2 pints vegetable stock
   (see page 77)
1 bay leaf

1 large onion, sliced
2 medium-sized carrots, diced
2 medium-sized potatoes, diced
Black pepper

Simmer the pearl barley in the stock, together with the bay leaf in a covered pan for about 1 hour. Add the vegetables and seasoning. Simmer for a further 30 minutes. Remove the bay leaf and serve.

# Minestrone soup

●          ◊         🌿🌿🌿

This is a very popular soup and traditional recipes can be improved by using wholewheat macaroni and reducing the amount of cheese, since hard cheeses like Cheddar tend to be high in fat content.

25 g/1 oz bacon
1 small leek
½ small carrot
½ small onion
½ small turnip
½ stick celery
900 ml/1½ pints vegetable stock
   (page 77)

Pepper
Bouquet garni
50 g/2 oz wholemeat macaroni
50 g/2 oz cabbage
50 g/2 oz cooked or frozen peas
25 g/1 oz grated cheese

Trim the bacon, cut into very small pieces and fry gently. Prepare the leek, carrot, onion, turnip and celery and chop finely. Soften the vegetables by heating them with the fried bacon for 5–10 minutes. Add the stock, seasoning, bouquet garni and the macaroni. Bring to the boil and simmer for about 45 minutes, stirring occasionally to prevent sticking. Chop the cabbage. Add together with the cooked or frozen peas. Cook for a further 5 minutes until the cabbage and peas are tender.

Serve with grated cheese sprinkled on top.


# Main courses

## Liver casserole

| 🌢🌢🌢🌢🌢🌢   ◊ | 🌿🌿 |
|---|---|

450 g/1 lb lamb's liver
50 g/2 oz wholemeal
   breadcrumbs
1 onion, minced finely
1 tbsp chopped parsley
1 level tsp mixed herbs

Pepper
Grated rind of ½ lemon
1 tbsp skimmed milk
225 g/8 oz can tomatoes,
   chopped

Preheat the oven to 180°C/350°F/Gas Mark 4.

Wash and trim the liver, removing any veins. Cut in slices and place in the bottom of a casserole. Make a stuffing by mixing together the breadcrumbs, onion, parsley, mixed herbs, pepper and lemon rind. Bind together with a little skimmed milk.

Cover the liver with the chopped tomatoes and spread the stuffing mixture on the top. Cover with tin foil. Cook in the centre of the oven for 30-45 minutes, until the liver is tender, removing the cover for the final 15 minutes to crisp up the top.


## Chicken casserole

| 🌢   | 🌿 |
|---|---|

Poultry is always preferable to red meats, as the fat content is lower. Removing the skin, where a lot of the fat is located, helps to reduce the fat further.

225 g/8 oz cooked chicken, diced
   and skin removed
100 g/4 oz mushrooms
6 whole spring onions
1 tbsp mixed dried peppers
225 g/8 oz tin tomatoes

4 tbsp skimmed milk
140 ml/¼ pint water
Black pepper
1 tbsp tomato purée
3 tsp cornflour

Place the prepared chicken in a casserole. Add the peeled mushrooms, chopped onions and dried peppers. Slice the tomatoes and
arrange on top (discarding the liquid). Mix the skimmed milk with
the water, pepper and tomato purée. Pour over the chicken and
vegetables. Cover the casserole and bake in a preheated oven at
220°C/425°F/Gas Mark 7 for about ¾ hour–1 hour. Remove from
the oven. Mix the cornflour with a little water. Add to the casserole
and return to the oven for a further 15 minutes.

# Quick chicken curry

Chicken is a low fat meat and using it in dishes like curry is also a
pleasant way to make it go further. The lentils in this dish increase
the protein and fibre content, making a filling and tasty dish for all
the family

1 medium onion, peeled and
   chopped
1 tbsp vegetable oil
1 tbsp curry powder
225 g/8 oz cooked chicken, diced

350 g/14 oz tin tomatoes
2 tbsp tomato purée
50 g/2 oz orange lentils
100 g/4 oz mushrooms

Fry onion in vegetable oil until softened. Add curry powder and fry
for a further minute, then add all other ingredients and stir. Bring to
the boil, cover and simmer steadily for about 40 minutes.

# Deep dish chicken and corn pie

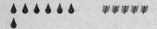

This pie could be made with any of the pastry recipes suggested in this book to increase the fibre content or lower the fat content of the pie.

1 small young roasting chicken
   or boiling fowl
2 onions
1 × 400 g/14 oz tin sweetcorn
50 g/2 oz margarine
100 g/4 oz tiny mushrooms

3 medium-sized, half-cooked
   potatoes
25 g/1 oz wholemeal flour

*Pastry*
160 g/6 oz wholemeal flour
3 tbsp skimmed milk powder
Water to mix

Put the chicken into a pan with the onions and enough water to cover. Simmer for about 45 minutes then drain, reserving the cooking liquid. Make the pastry by mixing the dry ingredients and adding enough water to make a dough; keep in a cool place. Drain the corn. Cut the chicken into neat pieces and toss it in the heated margarine. Add the mushrooms and half-cooked potatoes. Put the chicken and vegetables into a pie dish. Blend the flour with any fat in the pan. Cook for several minutes, then blend in 250 ml/½ pint of the reserved chicken stock. Bring to the boil and cook until thickened, pour over chicken and allow to cool.

Roll out the pastry, cover the top of the pie dish and bake at 220°C/425°F/Gas Mark 7 for about 45 minutes until the pastry is crisp and brown.

# Meat loaf

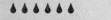

It is possible to vary the ingredients in this recipe to make the meat go further, for instance, by adding potato, mashed parsnip or swede. Even stewed apples can be added with success.

88

| 4 slices wholemeal bread | 1 medium onion, chopped fine |
| 340 g/12 oz minced beef | 1 carrot, grated finely |
| 1 egg | 2 tsp Italian seasoning |

Crumble the bread into crumbs, and mix together with all the other
ingredients. Spread in an ungreased loaf pan. Bake in the oven at
180°C/350°F/Gas Mark 4 for about 1 hour. Drain off the fat before
serving.

# Spaghetti bolognese

Minced meat usuall contains a lot of fat. Whenever you are making a
dish with mince it is helpful to cook the meat partly first, as in this
recipe, and drain off the fat before completing the dish.

| 2 tbsp oil | 225 g/8 oz tomatoes (canned or |
| 1 medium onion, chopped | fresh) |
| 1 stick celery, chopped | 1 tbsp tomato purée |
| 225 g/8 oz lean minced beef | 1 tbsp mixed herbs (Italian |
| 50 g/2 oz mushrooms | seasoning) |
| | Black pepper |

Heat the oil in a pan and gently fry the chopped onion and chopped
celery. Turn up the heat and add the meat. Stir continuously until
the meat begins to brown. Drain off the fat. Add the chopped
mushrooms, tomatoes (if fresh, remove the skins first) and tomato
purée. Boil for about 2 minutes. Add the herbs and pepper and turn
down the heat. Cook very gently, uncovered, for about 30 minutes.
Add more liquid if necessary.

# Lasagne

♦♦♦♦       🖻       ◊◊       ✹✹

225 g/8 oz lasagne
1 tbsp oil
1 onion, chopped
225 g/8 oz lean minced beef
500 g/16 oz tin tomatoes
Pepper
1 tbsp mixed herbs (Italian
   seasoning)

*Sauce*
25 g/1 oz margarine
1 tbsp cornflour
300 ml/½ pint skimmed milk
100 g/4 oz low fat cottage cheese
Salt and pepper

To make the sauce, warm the margarine in a small pan, add the
cornflour and stir until smooth. Add the milk and carry on stirring
until the sauce is smooth and thickened, then add the sieved cottage
cheese. Simmer for a minute or so and season lightly

   To cook the lasagne, bring a large uncovered pan of water to the
boil. Break each strip of lasagne into 10 cm/4 inch lengths and cook 4
or 5 of these pieces at a time. Drop them separately into the boiling
water and make sure that they do not stick together in the pan. Boil
until the pieces rise to the surface of the water, about 8 minutes.
After removing them rinse in cold water and spread out individually
on a damp tea towel. Cook all the lasagne in the same way.

   To make the meat sauce, heat the oil in a pan and fry the onion.
Add the meat and stir until it is well browned. Drain off surplus fat.
Add the tomatoes and seasoning, and simmer for about 30 minutes.

   Place alternate layers of lasagne, meat sauce and white sauce in a
casserole, ending with a layer of white sauce. Cook in the oven at
180°C/350°F/Gas Mark 4 for about 35 minutes.

# Chilli con carne

♦♦♦       🖻            ✹✹

This hot sauce goes well with rice which makes the meat go further
still.

340 g/12 oz lean minced beef
1 tbsp oil
1 large onion, chopped
1 clove garlic
1 green pepper, de-seeded and
    chopped

425 g/15 oz tin tomatoes
Pepper
1 level tsp chilli powder
1 tbsp vinegar
425 g/15 oz tin red kidney beans

Fry the beef in the fat until lightly browned. Add the onion, garlic and green pepper and fry for 5 minutes until soft. Drain off the fat. Stir in the tomatoes and add the pepper and chilli powder blended with the vinegar. Cover and simmer for about 1½ hours. Drain and rinse the red kidney beans. Add to the pan and cook for a further 15 minutes.

# Baked stuffed marrow

1 medium-sized marrow
2 onions
1 clove garlic (optional)
1 tbsp oil
225 g/8 oz minced beef
Thyme

Pepper
100 g/4 oz cooked brown rice
500 g/16 oz tin tomatoes
25 g/1 oz sultanas
Mixed herbs (Italian seasoning)

Heat a large pan of water and plunge the marrow in when boiling. Cook for 3 minutes, then remove from the pan. Slice off the top of the marrow lengthways about one third from the top to make a deep narrow receptacle with a shallow lid. Scoop out the seeds and membrane. If the space looks a little shallow, remove some pulp as well.

Chop the onions (and garlic if desired) and fry in the oil. Add the mince and fry till lightly browned. Drain off as much fat as possible. Add the thyme, pepper and cooked rice. Moisten the mixture with juice from the tomatoes and mix in the sultanas. Fill the scooped-out marrow with the mixture and fit on the lid, securing it with string or skewers. Boil up the tomatoes with a little pepper and mixed herbs till they can be mashed to a pulp. Place the marrow in a baking tin and pour the tomato mixture around. Bake in a moderate oven 180°C/350°F/Gas Mark 4 for 1 hour, or until the marrow is tender. Baste from time to time with the tomato sauce.

# Shepherd's pie

♦♦♦          ❦❦

By adding vegetables to the pie you can make a smaller amount of red meat go further.

| | |
|---|---|
| 2 carrots | 225 g/8 oz lean minced beef |
| 50 g/2 oz frozen peas | (cooked) |
| 1 onion | 450 g/1 lb mashed potato |
| 1 tbsp oil | (mashed to smooth |
| 140 ml/¼ pint water | consistency using a little of |
| 1 tsp Bisto | the cooking water) |

Wash and trim the carrots, slice them and cook with the peas. Chop the onion and fry gently in the oil. Drain off the oil. Add the water and Bisto and bring to the boil to form a rich gravy. Add the meat, carrots and peas. Turn into a pie dish. Pile on the mashed potato, smooth and heat through in the oven at 180°C/350°F/Gas Mark 4 for 20 minutes.

# Lamb kebabs

♦♦♦          🗐                    ❦❦❦

| | |
|---|---|
| 225 g/8 oz lean lamb | 100 g/4 oz button mushrooms |
| 1 medium green pepper | 8 small onions |
| 4 small tomatoes, halved | A little oil |

Remove all visible fat from lamb and cut into 2.5 cm/1 inch cubes. De-seed the pepper and cut into 2.5 cm/1 inch squares. Arrange

92

lamb pieces, tomatoes, mushrooms, green pepper squares and onions onto skewers. Brush with a little oil and place under a preheated grill for 10–12 minutes, turning frequently to ensure even cooking.

# Stuffed cabbage leaves

🌢🌢🌢　　　🌿🌿

This is a delicious way to use up any lamb left from a roast and if the quantity of meat available is rather smaller than the amount suggested here, the filling can be made up with a suitable vegetable like peas or diced carrots.

| | |
|---|---|
| 8 large cabbage leaves | Black pepper |
| 225 g/8 oz cooked lean lamb | 275 ml ½ pint stock (see page 77) |
| 100 g/4 oz cooked brown long-grain rice | 1 tbsp Worcestershire sauce |
| | 25 g/1 oz bran |
| 3 tbsp tomato purée | 2 tsp cornflour |
| 2 tsp mustard | |

Wash and trim the thick stalks of the cabbage leaves. Blanch in boiling water for 2 minutes then drain and dry. Mix together the lamb, rice, 2 tbsp of tomato purée, the mustard and pepper. Add a very little stock – just enough to moisten the mixture. Divide the lamb mixture between the cabbage leaves and roll them up to make little parcels, tucking in the sides neatly. Arrange the rolls, with the edge of each leaf underneath, in a shallow greased ovenproof dish. Pour the stock over, cover and bake at 180°C/350°F/Gas Mark 4 for 30 minutes. Pour off the stock, cover the dish and keep warm. Mix together the remaining tomato purée, the Worcestershire sauce, bran and cornflour. Gradually stir in the hot stock, transfer to a saucepan and bring to the boil, stirring well. Season with black pepper. Pour some of the sauce over the cabbage rolls before serving and serve the rest of the sauce separately.

# Italian veal casserole

♦ ♦ ♦                    ❦

If you don't like garlic this can easily be omitted or replaced by
onions.

340 g/12 oz lean veal
2 cloves of garlic, skinned and
   chopped
2 tbsp oil
Pepper

450 g/1 lb tomatoes, skinned and
   chopped
2 level tsp tomato purée
140 ml/¼ pint white wine
2 sprigs rosemary
1 strip of lemon rind

Trim off any visible fat and cut the meat into cubes. Fry the
chopped garlic in the oil until golden brown. Add the meat and
pepper and continue cooking until the meat is golden brown. Drain
off fat. Stir in the tomatoes, tomato purée, wine, rosemary and
lemon rind and just enough water to cover. Pour into a casserole,
cover tightly and cook in the centre of the oven at 180°C/350°F/Gas
Mark 4 for about 1 hour or until meat is tender.


# Fisherman's pie

❦

When making mashed potatoes, use a little of the cooking water to
obtain a smooth consistency.

450 g/1 lb cod
300 ml/½ pint skimmed milk
1 bay leaf

1 tbsp cornflour
1 tbsp chopped parsley
450 g/1 lb mashed potatoes

Simmer the fish in the milk with the bay leaf until it is tender. Strain
off the liquid and keep 300 ml/½ pint for the sauce. Remove the skin
and bones from the fish and flake. Place the reserved liquid in a
saucepan and bring to the boil; add the cornflour mixed to a smooth

paste with a little cold water. Stirring to keep the sauce smooth, add the chopped parsley. Mix the fish and the sauce and pour into a casserole. Spread the mashed potatoes over the top. Cook in a moderate oven 180°C/350°F/Gas Mark 4 for 25 minutes.

# Chinese baked fish

▲▲▲▲          ◇◇◇

750 g/1½ lb piece of cod/
   halibut/haddock (any thick,
   chunky fish)
3 spring onions

3 slices root ginger
2 tbsp soy sauce
1 tbsp corn oil

Clean fish and cut into four pieces. Chop the ginger into fine grains; chop the spring onions. Blend onions, ginger, soy sauce and vegetable oil in a bowl. Add fish and turn over so that it is completely coated in the mixture. Leave to marinate for about 1½ hours, turning occasionally. Preheat oven to 240°C/450°F/Gas Mark 7. Place fish in ovenproof dish and cover the top with a lid or foil. Bake for 10 minutes.

# Quick kedgeree

▲▲▲▲▲▲          🌾🌾

This recipe is a great one for a meal in a hurry and makes a very tasty and satisfying way of enjoying fish.

1 large onion
1 tbsp oil
1 tsp curry powder

450 g/1 lb cooked rice
200 g/7 oz tin tuna, drained and
   flaked

Slice the onion and fry gently in the oil. Add the curry powder and fry, stirring, for a few minutes. Add the cooked rice and tuna. Stir carefully to distribute the ingredients evenly, producing a warm, golden coloured dish. Do not overcook; the last step is only a mixing and reheating one.

# Cucumber relish

◊

This goes with kedgeree or any curry dish.

1 × 450 g/1 lb carton plain low fat yogurt
½ cucumber, peeled and coarsely grated

2 tbsp finely chopped fresh mint
¼ tsp cayenne pepper
Freshly ground black pepper

Put the yogurt in a bowl. Beat lightly with a fork or whisk until smooth and creamy. Add all the other ingredients and mix. Cover and refrigerate until ready to eat.

# Tuna noodle casserole

♦♦♦♦♦♦          ◊◊          ☙☙☙

A quick and satisfying meal, low in fat with plenty of fibre.

100 g/4 oz cut wholewheat macaroni
198 g/7 oz tin tuna
225 g/8 oz tin tomatoes
100 g/4 oz cottage cheese

2 tbsp plain yogurt
1 small onion, minced
75 g/3 oz wholemeal breadcrumbs

Cook and drain the macaroni. Add the tuna, well drained and flaked, the tomatoes, mashed, the cottage cheese, yogurt and onion. Mix well and pour into a greased casserole. Cover with breadcrumbs and bake at 180°C/350°F/Gas Mark 4 for about 30 minutes.

# Bean and cottage cheese flan

♦ ♦ ♦                    ◊ ◊                    ✹ ✹ ✹ ✹

*Pastry*
160 g/6 oz self-raising flour
3 tbsp skimmed milk powder
Water to mix

*Filling*
225 g/8 oz cottage cheese
2 eggs

75 g/3 oz cooked beans, any type
25 g/1 oz mushrooms
1 small onion, chopped
1 tsp dried tarragon
Black pepper
2 tomatoes
Chopped parsley

To make the pastry, mix together the flour and milk powder. Add enough water to make a dough. Roll out and line a flan tin.

Turn the cottage cheese into a basin and break up with a fork. Beat in the eggs and mix well. Stir in the beans. Wash the mushrooms and slice thinly. Reserve a few of the best mushroom slices for decoration. Soften the chopped onion and the mushrooms by simmering gently in a small amount of water. Drain well and add to the egg, cheese and bean mixture, together with the tarragon and pepper. Spoon into the flan case. Slice the tomatoes and arrange on the top with the mushroom slices.

Bake at 200°C/400°F/Gas Mark 6 for 15 minutes, then reduce the heat to 170°C/325°F/Gas Mark 3 for about 20 minutes until the filling is set. Garnish with chopped parsley.

# Asparagus flan

♦                    ◊                    ✹ ✹ ✹

This tasty flan, or our recipe for onion tart (page 98), makes a good alternative to the traditional quiche lorraine, which can be rather high in fat.

*Pastry*
160 g/6 oz wholemeal flour
3 tbsp skimmed milk powder
Water to mix

*Filling*
225 g/8 oz cooked asparagus (or
canned asparagus, drained)

1 egg
150 ml/¼ pint skimmed milk
1 tbsp chopped parsley
Black pepper
1 tbsp wholemeal flour
50 g/2 oz mushrooms, thinly
sliced, or 1 tomato, thinly
sliced

To make the pastry, mix together the flour and skimmed milk
powder. Add enough water to form a dough. Heat the oven to
190°C/375°F/Gas Mark 5. Roll out the pastry and line a 20 cm/8 inch
greased flan ring. Prick the base, line with foil and fill with dry beans.
Bake for 10 minutes. Remove foil and beans and bake for a further 5
minutes to dry the pastry base.

Chop the asparagus and place in the flan case. Beat together the egg
and milk, stir in the parsley, pepper and flour. Pour over the
asparagus and arrange the mushrooms or tomato slices in a pattern.
Bake for 30–35 minutes until the filling is set. Serve warm or cold.

# Onion tart

*Pastry*
160 g/6 oz self-raising flour
3 tbsp skimmed milk powder
Water to mix

*Filling*
900 g/2 lb onions
1–2 tbsp wholemeal flour
Pepper
1 egg
1 tbsp skimmed milk

To make pastry, mix the dry ingredients. Add sufficient water to
make a dough. Roll out and line a flan tin.

Peel and chop the onions and cook them over a low heat in just
enough water to prevent burning. When they are soft and tender,
take them off the heat and add just enough flour to bind them, with
the pepper, beaten egg and skimmed milk. Spread this thick mushy
onion mixture into the flan tin and bake in a fairly hot oven
(220°C/425°F/Gas Mark 7) for 20 minutes, then lower the heat and
continue cooking until the pastry is crisp and the top nicely
browned.

# Spanish omelette

♦♦       🄰       ◊       ❦❦❦❦❦

1 medium onion
1 tbsp oil
100 g/4 oz mushrooms
1 green pepper, chopped
450 g/1 lb cooked potatoes, diced

425 g/15 oz tin tomatoes, drained
  and chopped
3 eggs
150 ml/¼ pint skimmed milk
Pepper

Fry the sliced onion in the oil. Add the mushrooms and green pepper and cook for a few minutes, stirring. Add the potatoes and tomatoes, stir once carefully to distribute them but don't turn it into a great mush.

Beat the eggs, add the skimmed milk and pepper and pour over the vegetables in the pan. Cook slowly, shaking the pan occasionally. When the egg mixture shows signs of being cooked part of the way through, place the pan under the grill to cook the top side until golden brown.

Serve the omelette in wedges.

# Sausage rolls

♦♦♦♦♦♦♦       ◊       ❦❦❦
♦♦

No magic can make a dish with sausagemeat really low in fat, but this suggestion may help you to enjoy it as a treat and minimise the damage!

*Pastry*
160 g/6 oz wholemeal flour
3 tbsp skimmed milk powder
Water to mix

*Filling*
225 g/8 oz sausagemeat

50 g/2 oz oatmeal
1 cooking apple, peeled, cored
  and grated
Mixed herbs to taste
Pepper
A little skimmed milk

Make up the pastry by mixing the dry ingredients and adding enough water to make a soft dough. Roll out into a rectangle.

In a bowl, combine and blend the sausagemeat, oatmeal, apple and herbs. Divide the mixture into two. Form each portion into a 'snake' and place these on the pastry, so as to make two rows of sausage rolls, side by side. Dampen the edges of the pastry and fold over the sausagemeat to the middle; seal and cut the edges. Cut up into individual sausage rolls. Score the tops and brush with a little skimmed milk. Put into the oven at 240°C/475°F/Gas Mark 9, lowering the temperature immediately to 190°C/375°F/Gas Mark 5 and allowing time to cook through, about 30 minutes.

# Cornish pasties

| ♦ | ◊ | ❦❦ |
|---|---|---|

The traditional pasty provided the Cornish working man with a portable nutritious lunch. Too often its modern counterpart is too high in fat and salt – especially as the consumer is not going down the tin mines either! But they are so easy to make and so much healthier if you use this recipe.

*Pastry*
225 g/8 oz self-raising flour
4 tbsp skimmed milk powder
Water to mix

*Filling*
100 g/4 oz lean lamb

1 onion
1 carrot
2 potatoes
Pepper
1 tbsp water
Skimmed milk to glaze

Make the pastry by mixing together the dry ingredients and adding enough water to make a dough. Keep cool.

Trim off any visible fat from the meat and mince. Chop the onion and carrot and finely cut the potato into small dice. Mix together the meat, potato, carrot, onion, and pepper, adding the water to moisten. Divide the pastry into 4 portions and roll each into a round about 14 cm/5½ inches in diameter. Cut the edges neatly. Divide the meat filling and pile into the centre of each round. Dampen the edges of the pastry. Fold over, seal the edges together well and turn the pastry so that the sealed edges are over the top. Flute the edges and brush with skimmed milk. Bake for about 10 minutes or until the pastry begins to brown in a hot oven, 220°C/425°F/Gas Mark 7, then reduce the heat and allow time for the meat to cook at 180°C/350°F/Gas Mark 4 for a further 30 minutes.

# Pizza

♦ ♦        𝕊        ◊        ❦

3 level tsps active baking yeast
340 g/12 oz plain flour
225 g/8 oz tin tomatoes
4 spring onions
1 green pepper

100 g/4 oz mushrooms, thinly
  sliced
Mixed herbs (Italian seasoning)
100 g/4 oz Cheddar cheese,
  grated

Put the yeast in a few tablespoons of tepid water to dissolve for 10–15 minutes. Sift the flour into a warm basin. Make a well in the centre, pour in the yeast liquid, fold the flour over the top and mix well. Add enough tepid water to make a stiff dough. Move the dough on to a floured board and knead it for several minutes. After about 5 minutes it will change consistency, and become smooth, fine grained and lighter. Roll the dough into a ball, put it on a well-floured plate and cover it with a clean tea towel. Put it in a warm, draughtless place to rise for 2½–3 hours. By then the dough should have doubled in volume.

While this is happening, prepare the topping. Drain off the liquid and roughly chop the tomatoes. Chop the spring onions into rounds. De-seed the pepper and slice thinly.

Divide the dough into four pieces. Roll out each piece of dough to about ½ cm/¼ inch thick on a floured surface then transfer to non-stick baking sheets. Spread the surface quickly with tomato, onion, green pepper and mushrooms. Sprinkle with herbs, black pepper and finally cheese. Transfer quickly to a hot oven 230°C/450°F/Gas Mark 8 and bake for about 20 minutes. Eat at once or the base will become rubbery.

# Savoury filled pancakes

♦♦♦        ◊        ⅋⅋

*Pancake batter*
100 g/4 oz wholemeal flour
1 egg

300 ml/½ pint skimmed milk
1 tbsp oil

Put the flour into a basin. Add the egg and beat well. Gradually add the milk to make a smooth batter. Allow to stand in a cool place for about 30 minutes before use. Beat well immediately before using.
*To cook*: heat a small quantity of the oil in a frying pan. Pour in a little of the batter. Tip the pan so that the batter is evenly distributed. Turn over or toss when the surface has set and cook until lightly browned on the other side. Turn on to greaseproof paper and keep warm, until all the pancakes have been made in this way. Fill and serve.

*Suggested fillings*
• Tomato, onion and mixed herbs, simmered together. Cooled and cottage cheese added.
• Tuna and sweetcorn in white sauce made with skimmed milk and wholemeal flour.
• Chicken and sweetcorn in white sauce.

# Stuffed green peppers

♦♦       🧂🧂       ◊       ⅋⅋⅋⅋⅋

50 g/2 oz bacon, chopped
1 onion, chopped
100 g/4 oz mushrooms

200 g/8 oz cooked brown rice
Pepper
4 large green peppers

Fry the bacon and use the fat produced to fry the onion and mushrooms. Added the cooked rice and pepper. Cut the tops off the green peppers and remove the seeds. Cook in boiling water for 3 minutes and drain. Spoon the stuffing into the peppers, replace the tops and put into a baking dish with a little water. Bake for about 30–35 minutes at 190°C/350°F/Gas Mark 5.

# Broccoli casserole

♦♦♦♦                Ⓢ                ◊                ❦❦❦❦❦❦

225 g/8 oz wholemeal macaroni
450 g/1 lb broccoli
25 g/1 oz margarine
1 tbsp cornflour
300 ml/½ pint skimmed milk

50 g/2 oz low fat cottage cheese
Pepper
450 g/1 lb tomatoes
Parsley to garnish.

Cook the macaroni in plenty of boiling water. Drain. Trim the broccoli and cook in boiling water until just tender; drain. Melt the margarine, stir in the cornflour and cook gently for 1 minute, then add the milk and cottage cheese gradually to form a fairly thick sauce. Season.

Heat the oven to 200°C/400°F/Gas Mark 6. Slice the tomatoes thinly and reserve some slices for decoration. Cover the bottom of an ovenproof dish with a layer of tomato slices, cover with a layer of broccoli, then a layer of macaroni. Pour over a third of the sauce. Repeat these layers twice more, finishing with a layer of sauce. Decorate with the reserved slices of tomato. Bake for about 30 minutes; garnish with parsley before serving.

# Ratatouille

♦♦♦                Ⓢ                ❦

Commercial stock cubes may contribute rather a lot of sodium, so wherever possible it's better to use homemade stock. This recipe like many of the others in the book does not suggest seasoning with salt. This means that the consumers have more of a say in how much they are eating and can choose to add it later or not.

2 tbsp vegetable oil
1 medium-sized onion, skinned and sliced
1 clove garlic, crushed
1 medium-sized aubergine, sliced
1 green pepper, trimmed and sliced

2 medium-sized courgettes
4 tomatoes, skinned and sliced
250 ml/½ pint stock (see page 77)
Freshly ground pepper
2 tbsp chopped parsley

Heat the oil in a flameproof casserole. Fry the onion and garlic, then add the other prepared vegetables, stir well and fry for about 3 minutes. Add the stock and pepper. Cover and place in a moderate oven, 180°C/350°F/Gas Mark 4, for about 1 hour, until the vegetables are cooked but not mushy. Stir in parsley and serve.

# Pasta crunch

---

🍥🍥🍥🍥            ◊            ☙☙☙

---

100 g/4 oz wholemeal spaghetti rings
3 apples, thinly sliced
1 tbsp lemon juice

4 sticks celery, thinly sliced
3 tbsp raisins
3 tbsp low fat plain yogurt
Black pepper

Cook the pasta in plenty of boiling water for about 12 minutes. Do not allow it to become too soggy.

Core the apples, slice them thinly and toss them in the lemon juice. Stir in the celery, raisins and cooked pasta. Mix together with the yogurt and black pepper, blending thoroughly.

# Stuffed jacket potato

---

◊            ☙☙☙☙

---

A new way to enjoy those old favourites, baked potatoes. Of course, if you have a microwave, this can be a very quick as well as a satisfying meal in one.

| 4 large baking potatoes | 2 tsp chopped rosemary |
| 75 g/3 oz cottage cheese | 2 tsp chopped parsley |
| 225 g/8 oz cooked beans (haricot or red kidney) | 1 tsp grated lemon rind |
| | Black pepper |

Scrub the potatoes well, score their skins to prevent bursting and bake in a moderate oven, 180°C/350°F/Gas Mark 4, until cooked, 1–1½ hours depending on size. When the potatoes are soft, cut them in half and scoop the centres out carefully into a bowl, reserving the skins. Mash the potato in the bowl, add the cottage cheese, sieved, the beans, herbs, lemon rind and pepper. Mix well. Pack into the potato skins, mounding the filling. Reheat in the oven for about 10 minutes.

# Savoury leek pie

♦♦♦♦♦♦      🏚     ◊     🌾🌾🌾🌾🌾🌾

This is a tasty way to make the most of winter vegetables.

| 8 leeks | 75 g/3 oz grated cheese |
| 4 carrots | Parsley to garnish |
| 225 g/8 oz rolled oats | |

Thoroughly clean leeks and carrots. Cut leeks into 2.5 cm/1 inch lengths and slice carrots thinly. Cook gently in a small amount of water until just soft. Grease a pie dish, and add alternate layers of rolled oats, vegetables and grated cheese, repeating this sequence until the dish is full, ending with a layer of rolled oats and cheese. Pour in the remains of the vegetable water to moisten the rolled oats.

Place in a hot oven 220°C/425°F/Gas Mark 7 for 30 minutes, until the top is nicely browned. Sprinkle with parsley and serve hot.

# Crunchy parsnips

🌿🌿

450 g/1 lb parsnips
2 tbsp bran flakes
Parsley

Peel the parsnips and cut into pieces. Drop into boiling water which should just cover them. Boil gently until tender, about 30 minutes. Drain and mash. Place in a vegetable dish, level off the surface and sprinkle bran flakes over the top. Garnish with parsley.

# Saucy leeks

🗄🗄🗄          🌿🌿🌿🌿🌿

Vegetables don't have to be dull; the choice is not just between plain boiled or soaked in butter. With a recipe like this one you can add variety to the vegetables you serve.

4 medium-sized leeks

*Sauce*
396 g/14 oz tin tomatoes

1 medium onion, sliced
1 bouquet garni
Black pepper
Chopped parsley to garnish

Trim the leeks, cut them lengthways from the green and three-quarters of the way down, and wash carefuly between the leaves. Bring a large pan of water to the boil, drop in the leeks and boil until just beginning to get tender. Drain and run under cold water. While the leeks are cooking, make the sauce. Put all the ingredients in a pan and cook gently for about 20 minutes. Cool, remove the bouquet garni then liquidise for just a few seconds.

Lay the leeks neatly in an ovenproof dish, pour over the sauce, cover the dish and reheat at 190°C/375°F/Gas Mark 5 for about 30 minutes. Sprinkle with parsley before serving.

# Herring roe pâté

No need to spread fat on bread or crispbread when eating this pâté; just eat it by itself, spread thinly.

50 g/2 oz margarine
100 g/4 oz soft herring roes
2 tbsp chopped parsley

1 tbsp lemon juice
Pepper

Melt 25 g/1 oz of the margarine in a saucepan. Add the herring roes and fry gently for about 10 minutes. Soften the remaining margarine without melting it. Mash or liquidise the roes. Add the softened margarine, the chopped parsley, lemon juice and pepper. Mix well.

# Rice stuffing for roast chicken

It's nice to ring the changes on the accompaniments served with chicken and this recipe, based on a traditional Greek idea, is a way of adding a little more fibre. An alternative would be to use wholemeal rather than white bread in the more usual sage and onion stuffing. Slimmers are usually wary of nuts because of their high fat content, but it's worth remembering that they are high in polyunsaturates.

50 g/2 oz cooked brown rice
The liver of the chicken, chopped
1 small onion, skinned and chopped
50 g/2 oz raisins

50 g/2 oz almonds, blanched and chopped
2 level tbsp chopped parsley
1 tbsp corn oil
Freshly ground black pepper

Combine all ingredients and mix well together. Stuff bird as usual.

# Desserts and baking

## Banana surprise

8 bananas      ½ lemon
2 oranges      A few sultanas

Slice the bananas in half lengthways. Peel 1 orange and slice thinly. Grate the peel from the second orange and squeeze out the juice. Arrange slices of orange and banana in alternate layers in an ovenproof dish, finishing with a layer of oranges. Pour the orange juice and the juice of half a lemon over the lot. Sprinkle with a little lemon and orange peel and sultanas. Bake uncovered at 180°C/350°F/Gas Mark 4 until the bananas are soft and the fruits blended, about 20 minutes. (A dash of rum added before baking makes this a bit different for a special occasion.)

## Rhubarb crunch

Some fruits are naturally rather tart. But by combining the natural sweetness of dates with the rhubarb it's possible to avoid having to add sugar. Sugar would push up the calories without providing any fibre whatsoever.

450 g/1 lb fresh rhubarb      75 g/3 oz wholemeal flour
100 g/4 oz stoned chopped dates      75 g/3 oz rolled oats
     25 g/1 oz sugar

*Topping*      2 tbsp water
25 g/1 oz margarine

Clean and slice the rhubarb and add the chopped dates. Mix and place in an ovenproof dish. Rub the margarine into the wholemeal flour, add the oats and sugar, and mix thoroughly. Stir in water so that it is evenly distributed and the mixture has a crumbly texture. Cover the rhubarb with topping and bake at 190°C/375°F/Gas Mark 5 for 30–40 minutes.

# Orange sauce

🝪

This makes a very pleasant alternative to custard and is much lower in fat and sugar. You can vary the amount of cornflour to make the sauce as thick or thin as you like.

1 tbsp cornflour
250 ml/½ pt natural
    unsweetened orange juice
2 tbsp plain yogurt

Blend the cornflour to a smooth paste with a little of the orange juice. Place the rest of the orange in a small saucepan. Add the paste and bring to the boil, stirring continuously until thickened. Stir in the yogurt and serve.

# Rhubarb and orange mousse

🝪🝪🝪                ◊                🌿🌿🌿

450 g/1 lb rhubarb                15 g/½ oz gelatine
50 g/2 oz sugar                    2 egg whites
1 orange

Cut the rhubarb into chunks and cook gently in about 4 tablespoons of water with the sugar until tender. Grate the orange peel. Remove the skin of the orange and chop the flesh into small pieces. Dissolve the gelatine in 3 tablespoons of water over a gentle heat. Put the cooked rhubarb, the grated orange peel, the flesh of the orange and the gelatine in the blender. Blend on a low speed. Whisk the egg whites until stiff and fold into the fruit mixture. Leave in a cool place to set.

# Apricot and orange mousse

225 g/8 oz dried apricots
15 g/½ oz gelatine
1 tbsp unsweetened orange juice
3 egg whites

Soak the apricots overnight in 600 ml/1 pint water. Bring the fruit to the boil and simmer gently for about 1 hour or until very soft. Dissolve the gelatine in 3 tablespoons water over a very gentle heat. Put the apricots in the blender and blend until smooth. Add the orange juice and gelatine to the apricots. Whisk the egg whites until they are very stiff and fold in. Pour into individual dishes and leave in the refrigerator to set.

# Apple cobbler

1 kg/2 lb cooking apples          75 g/3 oz skimmed milk powder
½ tsp cinnamon                    Water to mix
75 g/3 oz self-raising flour      A little skimmed milk

Peel and core the apples and stew with the cinnamon. Turn the stewed apple into an ovenproof dish. Preheat the oven to 180°C/350°F/Gas Mark 4.
   Make the topping by mixing the flour, skimmed milk powder and

enough water to make a soft dough. Knead on a floured board and roll to 1 cm/½ inch thickness. Cut into rounds and arrange on top of the stewed apple. Brush with skimmed milk. Bake in the oven for 15-20 minutes or until nicely brown.

# Apple charlotte

This delicious, rich pudding can be accompanied by plain yogurt.

750 g/1½ lb cooking apples
Rind and juice ½ lemon
2 egg yolks

About 6 slices wholemeal bread
(8 mm/⅜ inch thick)

Bake the apples until soft and mash them. Mix with the grated lemon rind and juice and the egg yolks. Cut a round of bread to fit the base of a soufflé dish and a similar round for the top. Cut fingers of bread to fit exactly around the sides of the dish. Grease the dish and line with the pieces of bread. Put in the apple mixture and cover with the remaining slice of bread. Press down well with a saucer with weights on top and leave for about 1 hour. Bake at 190°C/375°F/Gas Mark 5 for 1–1½ hours. Turn on to a hot dish and serve.

# Blackberry and apple pie

A delicious blackberry and apple pie with pastry that won't add a lot of fat.

*Pastry*
160 g/6 oz self-raising flour
3 rounded tbsp skimmed milk
  powder
1 tsp caster sugar

*Filling*
225 g/8 oz blackberries
450 g/1 lb cooking apples

To make the pastry, sieve together all the dry ingredients and add enough water to form a dough. Roll out on a floured board and use half to line a 20 cm/8 inch pie plate. Wash and prepare the fruit, peeling and slicing the apples thinly. Pile into the pie plate. Cover with the remaining pastry, brush with liquid skimmed milk, and bake in a preheated oven at 190°C/375°F/Gas Mark 5 for 30 minutes.

# Peach Melba pie

---

🏠🏠🏠      ◇◇      🌾🌾🌾

---

225 g/8 oz self-raising flour      6 medium peaches
4 tbsp skimmed milk powder      300 g/10 oz fresh raspberries
Water to mix

Preheat the oven to 190°C/375°F/Gas Mark 5. Mix the flour, skimmed milk and enough water to make a soft dough. Roll out, and line a pie dish, reserving enough pastry for the pie top.

Wash the fruit. Remove the stones from the peaches and slice thinly. Mix the peach slices and raspberries and pile into the pie dish. Cover with the remaining pastry, seal the edges, make a slit in the pie crust for steam to escape and bake for approximately 25 minutes.

# Gooseberry fool

---

🏠      🌾🌾

---

3 tbsp natural yogurt
450 g/1 lb gooseberries
1 egg white

Cook the gooseberries in a very little water until soft, then purée. Stir in the yogurt when the fruit is cool. Beat the egg white and fold into the fruit mixture. Divide into serving dishes and chill.

# Satsuma delight

450 g/1 lb satsumas
600 ml/1 pint skimmed milk
25 g/1 oz custard powder

Peel the satsumas and set aside about a dozen segments. Make up
the custard. In the blender, whizz together the custard and satsumas. Pour into individual dishes. Allow to cool and decorate with
the reserved segments.


# Citrus circles

4 small oranges
2 grapefruit
½ teaspoon cinnamon
50 g/2 oz sultanas

Peel the fruit. Slice each one thinly crosswise to give a wheel
appearance. Arrange in a heatproof dish, interspersing orange and
grapefruit slices. Sprinkle the cinnamon and sultanas over the top.
Heat under the grill until the fruit is heated through and juice
bubbling up.

# Custard

♦♦♦           🍯🍯🍯           ◊

If made with skimmed milk

🍯🍯           ◊

Make to desired consistency with milk and custard powder. But try using skimmed milk, and halving the amount of sugar added at least.

# Tropical fruit salad

🍯🍯           🌾🌾🌾

1 tin lychees
1 small tin mangoes
1 small tin guavas
1 grapefruit

2 bananas
100 ml/4 fl oz unsweetened
    orange juice

Open the tins of tropical fruit. If they have been canned in syrup, place them in a sieve and rinse under the cold tap, discarding the syrup. Place in a bowl. Peel and roughly chop the grapefruit and add to the other fruit. Slice the bananas and add. Pour over the orange juice and mix all the fruit together carefully.

# Spicy bread pudding

♦           🍯🍯🍯🍯           ◊◊           🌾🌾🌾🌾

6 slices wholemeal bread
50 g/2 oz demerara sugar
2 teaspoons mixed spice

100 g/4 oz mixed dried fruit
600 ml/1 pint skimmed milk

Trim the crusts from the bread and cut into small pieces. Place in a bowl with two-thirds of the sugar, the spice and the fruit. Add the milk and mix thoroughly. Turn into an ovenproof dish and sprinkle with the remaining sugar. Place in a preheated oven, 200°C/400°F/Gas Mark 6, and bake for 30 minutes.

## Apple cinnamon yogurt

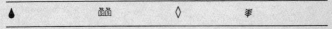

Commercial fruit-flavoured yogurts usually contain a lot of sugar. So try making your own combinations of fruit with natural low fat yogurt. A tablespoon of stewed apple and some cinnamon can transform a plain yogurt.

## Apricot raspberry yogurt

Combine pieces of different fruit in the same way with plain yogurt and you'll find you never want to go back to the sweetened blandness of shop-bought fruit yogurts.

## Spicy apple cake

1 large cooking apple
225 g/8 oz self-raising flour
3 tbsp skimmed milk powder
1 level tsp ginger
1 level tsp cinnamon

1 level tsp mixed spice
25 g/1 oz sugar
100 g/4 oz sultanas
Liquid skimmed milk to mix

Preheat the oven to 200°C/400°F/Gas Mark 6. Peel, core and slice the apple and simmer gently in a little water until soft. Set aside to cool. Mix together the flour, skimmed milk powder, spices, sugar, sultanas, cooked apple and a little liquid milk to make a soft consistency. Spoon into a 450 g/1 lb non-stick loaf tin and bake in the preheated oven. Reduce temperature after 20 minutes to 170°C/325°F/Gas Mark 3 for a further 20 minutes. Leave to cool in the tin for 30 minutes, then turn out on to a cooling tray.

# Honey bread

| 🧂🧂🧂 | ◊ | 🌾🌾 |
|---|---|---|

160 g/6 oz wholemeal flour  
½ tsp salt  
1 tbsp honey  
150 ml/5 fl oz skimmed milk  

½ tsp bicarbonate of soda  
50 g/2 oz sultanas  
50 g/2 oz raisins  

Preheat the oven to 170°C/325°F/Gas Mark 3. Place the flour and salt in a bowl and make a well in the centre. Gently melt the honey with half the milk. Dissolve the soda in the remaining milk. Mix these two. Pour into the flour and stir in the fruit. Turn into a 450 g/1 lb non-stick loaf pan. Bake for about 1½ hours until cooked through.

# Apricot relish

1 tsp = 🧂 🌾

225 g/8 oz dried apricots

Soak the apricots overnight. Drain and liquidise to a thick purée.

# Banana and raisin teabread

♦♦♦        🧂🧂🧂      ◊      🌾🌾

150 g/5 oz self-raising flour      50 g/2 oz brown sugar
75 g/3 oz wholemeal flour        3 bananas, mashed
1 tsp baking powder             75 g/3 oz margarine
Pinch salt                     100 g/4 oz dried mixed fruit
1 tsp mixed spice             2 eggs, lightly beaten

Preheat the oven to 180°C/350°F/Gas Mark 4. Grease two 450 g/1 lb loaf tins. Mix together the flours, baking powder, salt and mixed spice. Add the sugar, bananas, melted margarine, dried mixed fruit and eggs and beat for 3 minutes until smooth. Turn the mixture into the loaf tins and bake for 50 minutes to 1 hour, until cooked through. Stand the tins on a wire rack to cool slightly before turning out.

# Strawberry sponge cake

♦♦♦        🧂🧂🧂      🌾

As you can see from the score this is not something to eat every day, but if someone has a birthday in the strawberry season it would make a lovely choice.

2 eggs (size 3)             Pinch salt
50 g/2 oz caster sugar      225 g/8 oz fresh strawberries
50 g/2 oz plain flour        Icing sugar

Line two 18 cm/7 inch sandwich tins with greaseproof paper. Preheat the oven to 190°C/375°F/Gas Mark 5. Break the eggs into a bowl, add the caster sugar and beat with an electric beater until the mixture is light and thick.

Meanwhile, sift the flour and salt on to a piece of kitchen paper. When the egg and sugar mixture is ready sift the flour into it. Using a large metal spoon, lightly fold the flour into the mixture, working it as little as possible. Immediately the flour is distributed evenly, divide the mixture between the prepared tins. Tilt the tins to level the mixture rather than spreading it, to avoid breaking the air bubbles. Bake immediately in the preheated oven. (In order for the sponges to be light, it is essential that the mixture be handled gently and transferred to the oven quickly.) Bake for 20–25 minutes until the sponges are well risen, lightly golden and shrinking from the edges of the pan. Run a knife around the edge of the pan before turning out.

*Decorating*
Reserve 5 strawberries; mash the remainder and use this to sandwich together the two sponges. Dust the top of the cake very lightly with icing sugar. Then cut 4 strawberries in half and arrange at intervals round the cake, placing a whole strawberry in the middle. The cake should not be decorated too far in advance of eating as it may become a little soggy.

# Sunday tea cake

♦ ♦ ♦ ♦ ♦     &#x1f750;&#x1f750;&#x1f750;&#x1f750;&#x1f750;     ✹ ✹ ✹

The combination of oats and flour gives this cake an interesting texture as well as increasing its fibre content. The stewed apple helps to bind and sweeten the cake without adding fat or sugar. Cakes and biscuits are generally notorious for their hidden fat and sugar.

250 g/10 oz wholemeal flour
250 g/10 oz rolled oats
100 g/4 oz walnut pieces
150 g/6 oz raisins
75 g/3 oz coconut
300 g/12 oz stewed apple

1 tsp vanilla
Pinch of salt

*Filling*
150 g/6 oz stoned dates

Mix all the ingredients together to form a soft, slightly crumbly dough. Press or spread into two non-stick, 22.5 cm/9 inch round pans. Bake at 180°C/350°F/Gas Mark 4 for 40–50 minutes, until

118

golden brown. Let cool in the pans for 10 minutes, and then turn out for further cooling.

Make the filling by putting the dates into a saucepan with enough water to cover them and simmer for 10 minutes until soft. Mash to a paste, or whip in the blender, and spread on one of the cake rounds, covering with the other.

# Savoury scones

100 g/4 oz self-raising flour
100 g/4 oz wholemeal flour
50 g/2 oz margarine
50 g/2 oz strong cheese

Small pinch dry mustard
  powder
Approx. 4 fl oz skimmed milk

Preheat the oven to 240°C/475°F/Gas Mark 9. Mix the flours thoroughly, cut and rub in the fat. Mix in the cheese and mustard powder. Add enough skimmed milk to give a soft dough. Turn out on to a floured board and roll out to about 1 cm/½ inch thick. Cut out rounds with a 6 cm/2½ inch cutter and place on a non-stick baking sheet. Brush with skimmed milk and bake for about 10 minutes. Cool on a wire rack.

# Wholemeal bread

750 g/1½ lb wholemeal flour
1 level tbsp sugar
425 ml/¾ pint water, hand hot
  (i.e. 1 part boiling to 2 parts
  cold tap water)

3 level tsp dried active baking
  yeast
15 g/½ oz margarine or oil
2 level tsp salt

119

Put the flour in a large mixing bowl and stand in a warm place. Dissolve 1 teaspoon of the sugar in one third of the hand-hot water, then add the yeast and whisk. Stand the yeast mixture in a warm place until frothy, about 10 minutes. Rub the fat into the flour. Dissolve the rest of the sugar and salt in the hand-hot water and add this and the yeast to the flour. Mix until a smooth dough is formed and knead on a floured board until no longer sticky, about 5 minutes. Cover the dough and leave in a warm place for 30 minutes, until it doubles in size. Turn out and knead lightly. Divide in half. Knead each piece into a ball then shape and put into a greased 450g/1lb loaf tin. Preheat the oven to 230°C/450°F/Gas Mark 8. Cover the dough and leave in a warm place until the dough is 1 cm/½ inch above the top of the tins, about 30 minutes. Bake in the oven for approximately 30–35 minutes.

# The DIET 2000 Score Tables

A unique system to see at a glance what's in your food.

The following tables give symbol scores representing the average amounts of 'fat', 'fibre', 'sugar' and 'salt' in typical portions of a wide range of popular food items.

The symbols have the following values:

1 'fat' symbol       equals 2g of total fat
1 'fibre' symbol     equals 2g of dietary fibre
1 'sugar' symbol   equals 5g of simple sugars
1 'salt' symbol      equals 250mg of sodium

(Where necessary the symbol score for each item has been rounded up or down to the nearest whole symbol.)

## CEREAL PRODUCTS

Although you will see that some of the foods listed here contain fat, this is not principally of the saturated kind.

| | FAT | FIBRE | SUGAR | SALT |
|---|---|---|---|---|
| Barley ½oz (14g) raw-weight portion in thick soup | | ✹ | | |
| Bran 2 level tablespoons | | ✹ ✹ | | |
| Cornflour 1 level tablespoon | | | | |
| Custard powder 1 level tablespoon | | | | |
| Macaroni refined, 2oz (56g) dry weight | ♦ | ✹ | | |
| wholewheat, 2oz (56g) dry weight | ♦ | ✹ ✹ ✹ | | |

| Food | | | | |
|------|---|---|---|---|
| Oatmeal 1oz (28g) dry weight | ● | ✹ | | |
| Porridge 4oz (113g) serving | ● | ✹ | | ◇ ◇ ◇ |
| Rice refined, 2oz (56g) dry weight | | ✹ | | |
| brown, 2oz (56g) dry weight | | ✹ ✹ | | |
| Sago ½oz (14g) portion in serving of pudding | | | | |
| Semolina ½oz (14g) portion in serving of pudding | | | | |
| Spaghetti refined, 2oz (56g) dry weight | | ✹ | | |
| wholewheat, 2oz (56g) dry weight | | ✹ ✹ ✹ | | |
| in tomato sauce, 7oz (200g) | ● | ✹ | 🔲 | ◇ ◇ ◇ ◇ ◇ |
| Bread brown, 1¼oz (35g) 1 slice | | ✹ | | ◇ |
| Hovis, 1oz (28g) 1 slice | | ✹ | | ◇ |
| wholemeal, 1¼oz (35g) 1 slice | | ✹ ✹ | | ◇ |
| white, 1¼oz (35g) 1 slice | | ✹ | | ◇ |
| Bread roll brown crusty, average 2oz (56g) | ● | ✹ ✹ | | ◇ ◇ |

| | FAT | FIBRE | SUGAR | SALT |
|---|---|---|---|---|
| brown soft, average 2oz (56g) | ◖ ◖ | ✹ ✹ | | ◇ ◇ |
| white crusty, average 2oz (56g) | ◖ | ✹ | | ◇ ◇ |
| white soft, average 2oz (56g) | ◖ ◖ | ✹ | | ◇ ◇ |
| Crispbread rye type, 1 slice | | ✹ | | |

## *BREAKFAST CEREALS*

| | FAT | FIBRE | SUGAR | SALT |
|---|---|---|---|---|
| All Bran 1½oz (42g) average bowl | ◖ | ✹ ✹ ✹ ✹ ✹ ✹ | ▣ | ◇ ◇ ◇ |
| Corn Flakes 1oz (28g) average bowl | | ✹ ✹ | | ◇ ◇ |
| Grapenuts 1½oz (42g) average bowl | ◖ | ✹ ✹ | ▣ | ◇ |
| Muesli 2oz (56g) average bowl | ◖ ◖ | ✹ ✹ | ▣ ▣ ▣ | ◇ |
| Puffed Wheat ¾oz (21g) average bowl | | ✹ ✹ | | |
| Rice Krispies 1oz (28g) average bowl | | ✹ | | ◇ ◇ |
| Shredded Wheat ¾oz (21g) 1 Shredded Wheat | | ✹ ✹ | | |
| Special K 1oz (28g) average bowl | | ✹ | ▣ | ◇ |

| | FAT | FIBRE | SUGAR | SALT |
|---|---|---|---|---|
| Sugar Puffs 1oz (28g) average bowl | | ✹ | ▥▥▥ | |
| Weetabix 2 biscuits | ● | ✹ ✹ ✹ | | ◊ |

## *BISCUITS*

About half the fat in biscuits and cakes listed is of the saturated kind, so these are foods that need particular caution.

| | FAT | FIBRE | SUGAR | SALT |
|---|---|---|---|---|
| Digestive plain, 2 biscuits | ● ● | ✹ | ▥ | |
| chocolate, 2 biscuits | ● ● ● ● | ✹ | ▥▥ | ◊ |
| Ginger nut 2 biscuits | ● | | ▥ | |
| Custard cream 2 biscuits | ● ● ● | | ▥ | |
| Lincoln 2 biscuits | ● ● | | ▥ | |
| Rich tea 2 biscuits | ● ● | | ▥ | |
| Water biscuits | ● | | | |
| Fruit cake 3oz (85g) slice | ● ● ● ● ● ● | ✹ ✹ | ▥▥▥▥▥ ▥▥ | ◊ |
| Madeira 3oz (85g) slice | ● ● ● ● ● ● ● | ✹ | ▥▥▥▥▥ ▥ | ◊ ◊‹ |
| Sponge cake jam filled, 3oz (85g) slice | ● ● | ✹ | ▥▥▥▥▥ ▥▥▥ | ◊ ◊ |
| Doughnut 1 plain with jam | ● ● ● ● ● | | ▥▥ | ◊ |

124

| | FAT | FIBRE | SUGAR | SALT |
|---|---|---|---|---|
| **Eclairs** 1 with chocolate icing and cream filling | ● ● ● ● ● | | ▦ ▦ | ◇ |

## MILK AND DAIRY PRODUCTS

Milk and dairy products are an important source of saturated fats. About two thirds of the fat in whole milk and cheese is saturated and more than a third of the fat in an egg.

| | FAT | FIBRE | SUGAR | SALT |
|---|---|---|---|---|
| **Milk** fresh, 1 pint | ● ● ● ● ● ● ● ● ● ● ● ● | | ▦ ▦ ▦ ▦ ▦ | ◇ |
| milk in tea or coffee, 1 oz (28g) | ● | | | |
| skimmed, 1 pint | | | ▦ ▦ ▦ ▦ ▦ | ◇ |
| **Cream** single, 1 tablespoon | ● | | | |
| double, 1 tablespoon | ● ● ● | | | |
| **Camembert cheese** 1 oz (28g) | ● ● ● | | | ◇ ◇ |
| **Cottage cheese** 1 oz (28g) | ● | | | ◇ |
| **Cheddar cheese** | ● ● ● ● ● | | | ◇ |
| **Cream cheese** | ● ● ● ● ● ● ● | | | ◇ |
| **Danish blue** | ● ● ● ● | | | ◇ ◇ |
| **Edam type** | ● ● ● | | | ◇ |
| **Stilton cheese** 1 oz (28g) | ● ● ● ● ● ● | | | ◇ ◇ |
| **Yogurt** natural, 1 carton 5.3oz (150g) | ● | | ▦ ▦ | |

| | FAT | FIBRE | SUGAR | SALT |
|---|---|---|---|---|
| fruit, 1 carton 5.3oz (150g) | 💧 | | 🍬🍬🍬🍬🍬 | |
| hazelnut, 1 carton 5.3oz (150g) | 💧💧 | | 🍬🍬🍬🍬🍬 | |
| Egg, boiled or poached, 1 medium | 💧💧💧 | | | ◊ |
| fried, 1 medium | 💧💧💧💧💧 | | | ◊ |
| scrambled, 3½oz (100g) | 💧💧💧💧💧 💧💧💧💧💧 💧 | | | ◊◊◊ |
| Scotch egg, 1 | 💧💧💧💧💧 | | | ◊ |
| Cauliflower cheese 4oz (113g) serving | 💧💧💧💧 | 🌾 | | ◊ |
| Macaroni cheese 4oz (113g) serving | 💧💧💧💧💧💧 | 🌾 | | ◊◊ |
| Quiche Lorraine | 💧💧💧💧💧 💧💧💧💧💧 💧💧💧💧 | 🌾 | | ◊◊◊ |

## PUDDINGS

Many of these items are very high in fat as you can see, and about half the fat is saturated.

| | FAT | FIBRE | SUGAR | SALT |
|---|---|---|---|---|
| Apple crumble 4oz (113g) serving | 💧💧💧💧 | 🌾🌾 | 🍬🍬🍬🍬🍬 | ◊ |
| Cheesecake baked, 2oz (56g) serving | 💧💧💧💧💧 💧💧💧💧💧 | | 🍬🍬 | ◊ |
| Fruit pie 1 individual, pastry top and bottom | 💧💧💧💧💧 💧💧💧💧 | 🌾🌾 | 🍬🍬🍬🍬🍬 🍬🍬 | ◊ |
| Ice cream 2oz (56g) serving | 💧💧 | | 🍬🍬🍬 | |
| Custard made with milk and powder 2oz (56g) | 💧 | | 🍬 | |

| | FAT | FIBRE | SUGAR | SALT |
|---|---|---|---|---|
| Jelly 4oz (113g) serving | | | ▦ ▦ ▦ | |
| Lemon meringue pie 4oz (113g) serving | ◆ ◆ ◆ ◆ ◆ ◆ ◆ ◆ | ✾ | ▦ ▦ ▦ ▦ ▦ ▦ | ◇ |
| Rice pudding canned 4oz (113g) serving | ◆ | | ▦ ▦ | |
| Treacle tart 4oz (113g) serving | ◆ ◆ ◆ ◆ ◆ ◆ ◆ ◆ | ✾ | ▦ ▦ ▦ ▦ ▦ ▦ ▦ ▦ | ◇ ◇ |
| Trifle 4oz (113g) serving | ◆ ◆ ◆ | | ▦ ▦ ▦ ▦ | |
| Yorkshire pudding 2oz (56g) serving | ◆ ◆ ◆ | | | ◇ ◇ |

## MEAT AND MEAT DISHES

The fat content of meat and meat dishes is generally high, as you can see. About one-third to half of the fat in the different cuts of meat is saturated. Remember also that the fat you use for cooking can affect the final balance of saturated/unsaturated fats in a dish. So avoid using lard.

| | FAT | FIBRE | SUGAR | SALT |
|---|---|---|---|---|
| Bacon 1 back rasher, fried | ◆ ◆ ◆ ◆ ◆ | | | ◇ ◇ |
| 1 back rasher, grilled | ◆ | | | ◇ ◇ |
| 1 streaky rasher, fried | ◆ ◆ ◆ ◆ ◆ | | | ◇ ◇ |
| 1 streaky rasher, grilled | ◆ ◆ ◆ ◆ ◆ ◆ | | | ◇ ◇ |
| Gammon steak grilled, 1 slice 3½oz (99g) | ◆ ◆ ◆ ◆ ◆ ◆ | | | ◇ ◇ ◇ ◇ ◇ ◇ ◇ |
| Beef brisket boiled, 3 oz (85g) | ◆ ◆ ◆ ◆ ◆ ◆ ◆ ◆ ◆ ◆ | | | ◇ |

| Food | Fat | Salt |
|---|---|---|
| corned beef, 2oz (56g) | ● ● ● | ◇ ◇ |
| forerib roast, 3oz (85g) | ● ● ● ● ● ● ● ● ● ● ● ● | |
| mince stewed, 3oz (85g) | ● ● ● ● ● ● | ◇ |
| rumpsteak grilled, 8oz (226g) | ● ● ● ● ● ● ● ● ● ● ● ● ● ● ● | ◇ |
| rumpsteak fried, 8oz (226g) | ● ● ● ● ● ● ● ● ● ● ● ● ● ● ● | ◇ |
| silverside, salted boiled, 3oz (85g) | ● ● ● ● ● ● | ◇ ◇ ◇ |
| sirloin, roast, lean, 3oz (85g) | ● ● ● ● | |
| stewing steak, stewed, 3oz (85g) | ● ● ● ● ● | ◇ |
| topside, roast, lean, 3oz (85g) | ● ● | |

Lamb

| Food | Fat | Salt |
|---|---|---|
| lamb chop, grilled, lean and fat, 5oz (140g) | ● ● ● ● ● ● ● ● ● ● ● ● ● ● ● ● | |
| Lamb chop, grilled, lean only, 5oz (140g) | ● ● ● ● ● ● ● ● ● | |
| leg of lamb, roast, lean and fat, 3oz (85g) | ● ● ● ● ● ● ● | |
| breast of lamb, roast, lean and fat, 3oz (85g) | ● ● ● ● ● ● ● ● ● ● ● ● ● ● ● ● | |
| shoulder of lamb, roast, lean, 3oz (85g) | ● ● ● ● ● | |

| Food | Fat | Cholesterol |
|---|---|---|
| **Pork**<br>chop grilled, lean only, 7oz (200g) | ▲ ▲ ▲ ▲ ▲<br>▲ ▲ ▲ ▲ ▲ | |
| leg of pork, roast, lean and fat, 3oz (85g) | ▲ ▲ ▲ ▲ ▲<br>▲ ▲ ▲ | |
| leg of pork, roast, lean, 3oz (85g) | ▲ ▲ ▲ | |
| **Veal**<br>cutlet, fried, 3oz (85g) | ▲ ▲ ▲ | ◊ |
| fillet, roast, 3oz (85g) | ▲ ▲ ▲ ▲ ▲ | |
| **Chicken**<br>roast, light meat, no skin, 3oz (85g) | ▲ ▲ | |
| roast, leg, 3½oz (99g) | ▲ ▲ ▲ | |
| **Turkey**<br>roast, 3oz (85g) | ▲ ▲ | |
| **Rabbit**<br>stewed, weighed on the bone, 6oz (168g) | ▲ ▲ ▲ | |
| **Kidney**<br>lamb, fried, 2oz (56g) | ▲ ▲ | ◊ |
| ox, stewed, 2oz (56g) | ▲ ▲ | ◊ |
| **Liver**<br>lamb, fried, 4oz (113g) | ▲ ▲ ▲ ▲ ▲<br>▲ ▲ ▲ | ◊ |
| ox, stewed 3oz (85g) | ▲ ▲ ▲ ▲ | ◊ |
| **Tripe**<br>stewed, 6oz (170g) | ▲ ▲ ▲ ▲ | ◊ |
| **Beefburger**<br>frozen, fried 2oz (56g) | ▲ ▲ ▲ ▲ ▲ | ◊ ◊ |

| Food | Fat (drops) | Fibre | Diamonds |
|---|---|---|---|
| **Hamburger in bun** 1 regular | ● ● ● ● ● | ✹ | ◇ ◇ |
| **Beef stew** 4oz (113g) serving | ● ● ● ● | ✹ | ◇ ◇ |
| **Black pudding** 3oz (85g) | ● ● ● ● ● ● ● ● ● | | ◇ ◇ ◇ ◇ |
| **Bolognese sauce** 4oz (113g) serving | ● ● ● ● ● ● | | ◇ ◇ |
| **Brawn** 2oz (56g) | ● ● ● | | ◇ ◇ |
| **Cornish pasty** 1 pasty, 6.7oz (190g) | ● ● ● ● ● ● ● ● ● ● ● ● ● ● ● ● ● ● ● ● | ✹ | ◇ ◇ ◇ ◇ |
| **Curried meat** 4 oz (113g) serving | ● ● ● ● ● ● | ✹ | ◇ ◇ |
| **Faggots** 3oz (85g) | ● ● ● ● ● ● ● ● | | ◇ ◇ ◇ |
| **Frankfurters** 1 2oz (56g) | ● ● ● ● ● ● ● | | ◇ ◇ |
| **Haggis** 3oz (85g) | ● ● ● ● ● ● ● ● ● | | ◇ ◇ ◇ |
| **Ham** 2 slices 2oz (56g) | ● | | ◇ ◇ ◇ |
| **Ham & pork chopped** 3 oz (85g) | ● ● ● ● ● ● ● ● ● ● | | ◇ ◇ ◇ ◇ |
| **Liver sausage** 1oz (28g) enough to fill 1 sandwich | ● ● ● ● | | ◇ |

| Food | Fat | | |
|---|---|---|---|
| **Luncheon meat**<br>3oz (85g) | ◊ ◊ ◊ ◊ ◊ ◊ ◊ ◊ ◊ ◊ ◊ | | ◇ ◇ ◇ ◇ |
| **Moussaka**<br>6oz (170g) serving | ◊ ◊ ◊ ◊ ◊ ◊ ◊ ◊ ◊ ◊ ◊ | ✺ | ◇ ◇ |
| **Pork pie**<br>1 individual 5oz<br>(142g) | ◊ ◊ ◊ ◊ ◊ ◊ ◊ ◊ ◊ ◊ ◊ ◊ ◊ ◊ ◊ ◊ ◊ ◊ | ✺ | ◇ ◇ ◇ ◇ |
| **Salami**<br>1 oz (28oz) | ◊ ◊ ◊ ◊ ◊ ◊ | | ◇ ◇ |
| **Sausages**<br>beef, fried, 1 2oz<br>(56g) | ◊ ◊ ◊ ◊ ◊ | | ◇ ◇ ◇ |
| beef, grilled, 1 2oz<br>(56g) | ◊ ◊ ◊ ◊ ◊ | | ◇ ◇ ◇ |
| pork, fried, 1 2oz<br>(56g) | ◊ ◊ ◊ ◊ ◊ ◊ ◊ | | ◇ ◇ ◇ |
| pork, grilled, 1 2oz<br>(56g) | ◊ ◊ ◊ ◊ ◊ ◊ | | ◇ ◇ ◇ |
| **Sausage roll**<br>flaky pastry, 1 roll<br>2oz (56g) | ◊ ◊ ◊ ◊ ◊ ◊ ◊ ◊ ◊ ◊ | ✺ | ◇ ◇ |
| **Shepherd's pie**<br>6oz (170g) serving | ◊ ◊ ◊ ◊ ◊ | ✺ | ◇ ◇ ◇ |
| **Steak & kidney pie**<br>1 individual pie 5oz<br>(142oz) | ◊ ◊ ◊ ◊ ◊ ◊ ◊ ◊ ◊ ◊ ◊ ◊ ◊ ◊ ◊ | ✺ | ◇ ◇ ◇ |
| **Tongue**<br>2oz (56g) | ◊ ◊ ◊ ◊ ◊ | | ◇ ◇ ◇ |

131

# FISH & FISH DISHES

These are generally lower in fat than the meat dishes, and the fat is much less likely to be saturated.

| | FAT | FIBRE | SUGAR | SALT |
|---|---|---|---|---|
| Cockles<br>2oz (56g) boiled in<br>salt water | | | | ◊◊◊◊<br>◊◊◊ |
| Cod<br>steamed, 6oz (170g)<br>portion | ◆ | | | ◊ |
| fried in batter, 6oz<br>(170g) portion | ◆◆◆◆◆<br>◆◆◆◆ | | | ◊ |
| Crab<br>1½oz (42g) tin | | | | ◊ |
| Fishcakes<br>1 fishcake, fried | ◆◆◆ | | | ◊ |
| Fish fingers<br>1 fish finger, fried | ◆◆◆ | | | ◊ |
| Fish paste<br>1oz (28g) | ◆ | | | ◊ |
| Haddock<br>fried in<br>breadcrumbs, 6oz<br>(170g) portion | ◆◆◆◆◆<br>◆◆ | | | ◊ |
| steamed, 6oz (170g)<br>portion | ◆ | | | ◊ |
| Lemon sole<br>fried in<br>breadcrumbs,<br>average fish 4oz<br>(113g) | ◆◆◆◆◆<br>◆◆ | | | ◊ |
| Plaice<br>fried in batter, 6oz<br>(170g) portion | ◆◆◆◆◆<br>◆◆◆◆◆<br>◆◆◆◆◆ | ✿ | | ◊◊ |
| steamed, 6oz (170g)<br>portion | ◆◆ | | | ◊◊ |

| Food | | |
|---|---|---|
| Herring<br>grilled, average fish<br>5oz (142g) | ♦ ♦ ♦ ♦ ♦<br>♦ ♦ ♦ ♦ | ◊ |
| Kipper<br>grilled, average fish<br>6oz (170g) | ♦ ♦ ♦ ♦ ♦ | ◊ ◊ ◊ |
| Mackerel<br>fried, average fish<br>6oz (170g) | ♦ ♦ ♦ ♦ ♦<br>♦ ♦ ♦ ♦ | ◊ |
| Mussels<br>boiled in water, 2oz<br>(56g) | ♦ | ◊ |
| Pilchards<br>tinned in tomato<br>sauce, 1 pilchard<br>2½oz (70g) | ♦ ♦ | ◊ |
| Prawns<br>2oz (56g) serving | ♦ | ◊ ◊ ◊ |
| Salmon<br>tinned 3oz (85g)<br>serving | ♦ ♦ ♦ | ◊ ◊ |
| Salmon<br>smoked, 1oz (28g)<br>serving | ♦ | ◊ ◊ |
| Sardines<br>in oil, 2oz (56g) | ♦ ♦ ♦ ♦ | ◊ ◊ |
| Sardines<br>tinned in tomato<br>sauce, 2oz (56g) | ♦ ♦ ♦ | ◊ ◊ |
| Scampi<br>fried, 3oz (85g)<br>serving | ♦ ♦ ♦ ♦ ♦ ❀<br>♦ ♦ | ◊ |
| Skate<br>fried in batter, 6oz<br>(170g) serving | ♦ ♦ ♦ ♦ ♦<br>♦ ♦ ♦ ♦ ♦ | ◊ |
| Trout<br>6oz (170g) serving | ♦ ♦ ♦ ♦ | ◊ |

# VEGETABLES

Basically these are fat free. If you are going to add fat when mashing them, or if you decide to fry, use a fat or oil that is less saturated.

| | FAT | FIBRE | SUGAR | SALT |
|---|---|---|---|---|
| Asparagus 1 spear | | | | |
| Aubergine average size 7oz (198g) | | 🌿🌿🌿 | 🧂 | |
| Beans French, 3oz (113g) serving | | 🌿🌿 | | |
| runner, boiled, 3oz (113g) serving | | 🌿🌿 | | |
| broad, boiled, 3oz (113g) serving | | 🌿🌿🌿 | | |
| butter, boiled, 3oz (113g) serving | | 🌿🌿🌿 | | |
| haricot, uncooked, 1oz (28g) | | 🌿🌿🌿🌿 | | |
| baked, tinned in tomato sauce, 3oz (113g) serving | | 🌿🌿🌿🌿 | 🧂 | ◊ ◊ |
| red kidney, uncooked, 1oz (28g) | | 🌿🌿🌿 | | |
| Beansprouts 2oz (56g) serving | | 🌿 | | |
| Beetroot boiled, 2oz (56g) serving | | 🌿 | 🧂 | |
| Brussels sprouts 4oz (113g) serving | | 🌿🌿 | | |
| Cabbage spring, boiled, 4oz (113g) serving | | 🌿🌿 | | |

134

| Food | | | |
|---|---|---|---|
| white, raw, 3oz (85g) | ✹ ✹ | | |
| winter, boiled, 4oz (113g) | ✹ ✹ | | |
| Carrots raw, 2oz (56g) | ✹ | | |
| boiled, 4oz (113g) serving | ✹ ✹ | ▥ | |
| tinned, 4oz (113g) serving | ✹ ✹ | ▥ | ◊ |
| Cauliflower boiled, 4oz (113g) serving | ✹ | | |
| Celery raw, large stick, 2oz (56g) | ✹ | | ◊ |
| Chicory raw, 1oz (28g) serving | | | |
| Cucumber 2oz (56g) serving | | | |
| Endive 2 oz (56g) serving | ✹ | | |
| Leeks boiled, 4oz (113g) serving | ✹ ✹ ✹ | ▥ | |
| Lentils uncooked, 1½oz (42g) | ✹ ✹ ✹ | | |
| Lettuce 1 oz (28g) | | | |
| Marrow boiled, 4oz (113g) serving | ✹ | | |

| Food | Fat (droplets) | Fibre (flowers) | Other | Diamonds |
|---|---|---|---|---|
| **Mushrooms** raw, 2oz (56g) serving | | ❀ | | |
| fried, 2oz (56g) serving | ♦ ♦ ♦ ♦ ♦ ♦ | ❀ ❀ | | |
| **Onions** fried, 2oz (56g) serving | ♦ ♦ ♦ ♦ ♦ ♦ ♦ ♦ ♦ | ❀ ❀ | | |
| spring, raw, ½oz (14g) salad serving | | | | |
| **Parsnips** boiled, 4oz (113g) serving | | ❀ ❀ | 🗊 | |
| **Peas** frozen, boiled, 4oz (113g) serving | | ❀ ❀ ❀ ❀ ❀ ❀ | | |
| garden, tinned, 4oz (113g) serving | | ❀ ❀ ❀ ❀ | 🗊 | ◊ |
| processed, tinned, 4oz (113g) serving | | ❀ ❀ ❀ ❀ ❀ | | ◊ ◊ |
| dried, uncooked, 1½oz (42g) | | ❀ ❀ ❀ ❀ | | |
| split, dried, 2oz (56g) | | ❀ ❀ ❀ ❀ | | |
| **Chick peas** raw, 1oz (28g) | | ❀ ❀ | | |
| **Pepper** green, raw, 1oz (28g) salad serving | | | | |
| **Potatoes** old, boiled, 4oz (113g) serving | | ❀ | | |
| new, boiled, 4oz (113g) serving | | ❀ | | |
| mashed, 4oz (113g) serving | ♦ ♦ ♦ | ❀ | | |

| Food | | | |
|---|---|---|---|
| baked with skin, 7oz (198g) | | ✹ ✹ | |
| roast, 2oz (56g) | ● | | |
| chips, 4oz (113g) serving | ● ● ● ● ● ● | ✹ | |
| crisps, small packet | ● ● ● ● ● | ✹ ✹ | |
| Spinach boiled, 4oz (113g) serving | | ✹ ✹ ✹ ✹ | ◇ |
| Spring greens 4oz (113g) serving | | ✹ ✹ | |
| Swedes boiled, 4oz (113g) serving | | ✹ ✹ | ▣ |
| Sweetcorn tinned, 3oz (85g) serving | | ✹ ✹ | ▣ ◇ |
| on the cob, 3oz (85g) | ● | ✹ ✹ | |
| Tomatoes 1 fresh tomato, 2oz (56g) | | ✹ | |
| fried tomatoes, 2oz (56g) | ● ● | ✹ | |
| tinned, 4oz (113g) serving | | ✹ | |
| Turnips boiled, 4oz (113g) serving | | ✹ ✹ | |
| Watercress 1oz (28g) salad serving | | ✹ | |

# *FRUIT*

Apart from avocado pears, you won't find any fat in fruit. Even the
avocado is rich in predominantly unsaturated fat.

| | FAT | FIBRE | SUGAR | SALT |
|---|---|---|---|---|
| **Apple** eating, average-sized fruit, 5oz (142g) | | 🌾 | 🧂 🧂 | |
| cooking, baked with skin, 8oz (227g) | | 🌾 🌾 | 🧂 🧂 🧂 🧂 | |
| cooking, stewed without sugar, 6oz (170g) | | 🌾 🌾 | 🧂 🧂 🧂 | |
| **Apricots** one average fruit, 1oz (28g) | | 🌾 | | |
| stoned, stewed without sugar, 6oz (170g) | | 🌾 🌾 | 🧂 🧂 | |
| dried, stoned, stewed without sugar, 4oz (113g) | | 🌾 🌾 🌾 🌾 🌾 | 🧂 🧂 🧂 | |
| canned, 4oz (113g) | | 🌾 | 🧂 🧂 🧂 🧂 🧂 🧂 | |
| **Avocado pear** ½ an avocado, 3½oz (99g) | 💧 💧 💧 💧 💧 💧 💧 💧 💧 💧 💧 | 🌾 | | |
| **Banana** one average-sized fruit, 6oz (170g) | | 🌾 🌾 🌾 | 🧂 🧂 🧂 🧂 🧂 | |
| **Blackberries** stewed without sugar, 4oz (113g) | | 🌾 🌾 🌾 🌾 | 🧂 | |

| Food | | |
|---|---|---|
| **Blackcurrants** stewed without sugar, 4oz (113g) serving | 🌾🌾🌾🌾 | 🍯 |
| **Cherries** eating, 4oz (113g) | 🌾 | 🍯🍯 |
| glacé, 4oz (113g) | 🌾 | 🍯🍯🍯🍯🍯 ◊<br>🍯🍯🍯🍯🍯<br>🍯🍯 |
| **Currants** dried, ½oz (14g) | 🌾 | 🍯🍯 |
| **Damsons** stewed without sugar, 4oz (113g) serving | 🌾🌾 | 🍯🍯 |
| **Dates** dried, no stones, 2oz (56g) | 🌾🌾🌾 | 🍯🍯🍯🍯🍯<br>🍯🍯 |
| **Figs** fresh raw, 1oz (28g) 1 average-sized fruit | 🌾 | |
| dried, 2oz (56g) 2–3 figs | 🌾🌾🌾🌾🌾 | 🍯🍯🍯🍯🍯<br>🍯 |
| **Fruit pie filling** tinned 1 can 10½oz (300g) | 🌾🌾🌾 | 🍯🍯🍯🍯🍯 ◊<br>🍯🍯🍯🍯🍯<br>🍯🍯🍯🍯 |
| **Gooseberries** stewed without sugar 4oz (113g) serving | 🌾🌾 | 🍯 |
| **Grapes** black, 4oz (113g) | | 🍯🍯🍯 |
| green, 4oz (113g) | 🌾 | 🍯🍯🍯 |
| **Grapefruit** ½ fresh fruit | 🌾 | 🍯 |

| Food | | |
|---|---|---|
| canned in syrup, 4oz (113g) serving | | 🛍️🛍️🛍️ |
| Greengages stewed without sugar, 4oz (113g) serving | 🌾 | 🛍️🛍️ |
| Guavas tinned, 4oz (113g) serving | 🌾 | 🛍️🛍️🛍️ |
| Loganberries stewed without sugar, 4oz (113g) serving | 🌾🌾🌾 | 🛍️ |
| tinned, 4oz (113g) serving | 🌾🌾🌾 | 🛍️🛍️🛍️ |
| Lychees tinned, 4oz (113g) serving | | 🛍️🛍️🛍️🛍️ |
| Mandarin oranges tinned, 4oz (113g) serving | | 🛍️🛍️🛍️ |
| Mangoes tinned, 4oz (113g) serving | 🌾 | 🛍️🛍️🛍️🛍️🛍️ |
| Melon cantaloupe, 8oz (227g) serving | 🌾 | 🛍️ |
| yellow/honeydew, 8oz (227g) serving | 🌾 | 🛍️🛍️ |
| watermelon, 8oz (227g) serving | 🌾 | 🛍️ |
| Mulberries 4oz (113g) serving | 🌾 | 🛍️🛍️ |
| Nectarines 1 average-sized fruit, 5oz (142g) | 🌾🌾 | 🛍️🛍️🛍️ |

| Food | | |
|---|---|---|
| Olives, 1 olive | | ◊ |
| Oranges raw, 1 average-sized fruit | 🌾 | 🏺🏺 |
| Passion fruit raw, 1 average-sized fruit | 🌾🌾🌾 | |
| Paw-paw tinned, 4oz (113g) serving | | 🏺🏺🏺🏺 |
| Peach fresh, 1 whole fruit | 🌾 | 🏺🏺 |
| Peach tinned, 4oz (113g) serving | 🌾 | 🏺🏺🏺🏺🏺 |
| Pear eating, 1 average-size fruit | 🌾 | 🏺🏺 |
| Pear cooking, stewed without sugar, 4oz (113g) serving | 🌾🌾 | 🏺🏺 |
| Pear tinned in syrup, 4oz (113g) serving | 🌾 | 🏺🏺🏺🏺 |
| Pineapple fresh, 1 slice without skin | 🌾 | 🏺 |
| Pineapple tinned in syrup, 4oz (113g) serving | 🌾 | 🏺🏺🏺🏺 |
| Plums fresh dessert, 1 average fruit | 🌾 | 🏺 |
| Plums stewed, without sugar, with stones, 6oz (170g) | 🌾🌾 | 🏺🏺 |
| Prunes stewed, without sugar, 4oz (113g) serving | 🌾🌾🌾🌾🌾 | 🏺🏺🏺🏺 |

| | FIBRE | SUGAR |
|---|---|---|
| Raisins<br>dried, ½oz (14g)<br>serving, e.g. with<br>cereal | ✹ | 🍯🍯 |
| Raspberries<br>raw, 4oz (113g)<br>serving | ✹ ✹ ✹ ✹ | 🍯 |
| stewed, without<br>sugar, 4oz (113g)<br>serving | ✹ ✹ ✹ ✹ | 🍯 |
| tinned, 4oz (113g)<br>serving | ✹ ✹ ✹ | 🍯🍯🍯🍯🍯 |
| Redcurrants<br>stewed, without<br>sugar, 4oz (113g)<br>serving | ✹ ✹ ✹ ✹ | 🍯 |
| Rhubarb<br>stewed, without<br>sugar, 4oz (113g)<br>serving | ✹ | |
| Strawberries<br>fresh, 4oz (113g)<br>serving | ✹ | 🍯 |
| Sultanas<br>dried, ½oz (14g)<br>serving, e.g. with<br>cereal | ✹ | 🍯🍯 |
| Tangerines<br>1 average fruit | ✹ | 🍯 |

## NUTS

Apart from coconut, which is a rich source of saturated fats, most nuts contain predominantly unsaturated fats.

| | FAT | FIBRE | SUGAR | SALT |
|---|---|---|---|---|
| Almonds<br>1oz (28g) | 💧💧💧💧💧💧💧💧 | ✹ ✹ | | |

| | FAT | FIBRE | SUGAR | SALT |
|---|---|---|---|---|
| Brazil nuts<br>1oz (28g) | 9 droplets | 2 | | |
| Chestnuts<br>shelled, 1oz (28g) | | 1 | | |
| Hazelnuts<br>shelled, 1oz (28g) | 6 droplets | 1 | | |
| Coconut<br>fresh, 1oz (28g) | 6 droplets | 2 | | |
| dessicated, 1oz (28g) | 10 droplets | 3 | | |
| Peanuts<br>fresh, 1oz (28g) | 8 droplets | 1 | | |
| roasted & salted, 1 small packet | 8 droplets | 1 | | 1 |
| Peanut butter<br>½oz (14g), enough for 1 sandwich | 3 droplets | 1 | | |
| Walnuts<br>shelled, 1oz (28g) | 8 droplets | 1 | | |

## SWEET THINGS

| | FAT | FIBRE | SUGAR | SALT |
|---|---|---|---|---|
| Black treacle<br>1 level tablespoon | | | 3 | |
| Bounty bar<br>1 bar | 8 droplets | | 6 | |
| Chocolate<br>milk, small bar | 9 droplets | | 6 | |
| plain, small bar | 9 droplets | | 6 | |

143

| Food | FAT | FIBRE | SUGAR | SALT |
|---|---|---|---|---|
| Fruit gums 1 tube | | | ▦▦▦ | |
| Golden syrup 1 level tablespoon | | | ▦▦▦ | |
| Honey 1 level teaspoon | | | ▦ | |
| Jam 1 level teaspoon | | | ▦ | |
| Lemon curd 1 level teaspoon | | | ▦ | |
| Marmalade 1 level teaspoon | | | ▦ | |
| Mars bar 1 bar | ●●●●● ● | | ▦▦▦▦▦ ▦▦▦▦ | |
| Marzipan 1oz (28g) | ●●● | 🌾 | ▦▦▦ | |
| Mincemeat 1oz (28g) | ● | | ▦▦▦ | |
| Sugar demarara, 1 level teaspoon | | | ▦ | |
| white, 1 level teaspoon | | | ▦ | |

## DRINKS

| Drink | FAT | FIBRE | SUGAR | SALT |
|---|---|---|---|---|
| Coca cola 1 can | | | ▦▦▦▦▦ ▦▦ | |
| Ginger ale 4oz (113g) mixer | | | ▦▦ | |
| Grapefruit juice tinned, sweetened, 4oz (113g) serving | | | ▦▦ | |

| | FAT | FIBRE | SUGAR | SALT |
|---|---|---|---|---|
| **Lemonade** <br> 8oz (226g) serving | | | ▦▦▦ | |
| **Lucozade** <br> 8oz (226g) serving | | | ▦▦▦▦ | |
| **Milkshake** <br> vanilla, thick | ●●●● | | ▦▦▦▦▦ ◊ <br> ▦▦▦▦▦ <br> ▦▦ | |
| **Orange squash** <br> 1oz (28g) undiluted | | | ▦▦ | |
| **Orange juice** <br> fresh, 4oz (113g) serving | | | ▦▦ | |
| tinned, unsweetened, 4oz (113g) serving | | | ▦▦ | |
| **Pineapple juice** <br> tinned, 4oz (113g) serving | | | ▦▦▦ | |
| **Ribena** <br> 1oz (28g) undiluted | | | ▦▦▦ | |
| **Tomato juice** <br> tinned, 4oz (113g) serving | | | ▦ | ◊ |
| **Tonic water** <br> 4oz (113g) mixer | | | ▦▦ | |

## ALCOHOLIC DRINKS

| | FAT | FIBRE | SUGAR | SALT |
|---|---|---|---|---|
| **Beer** <br> brown ale, ½ pint | | | ▦▦ | |
| draught bitter, ½ pint | | | ▦ | |
| draught mild, ½ pint | | | ▦ | |
| lager, ½ pint | | | ▦ | |

| | SUGAR |
|---|---|
| pale ale, ½ pint | ▯ |
| stout, ½ pint | ▯▯ |
| Cider<br>dry, ½ pint | ▯ |
| sweet, ½ pint | ▯▯ |
| Wines<br>red, 1 glass | |
| rosé, 1 glass | ▯ |
| white dry, 1 glass | |
| white sweet, 1 glass | ▯ |
| white sparkling, 1 glass | |
| Port<br>1 glass | ▯ |
| Sherry<br>dry, 1 glass | |
| medium, 1 glass | |
| sweet, 1 glass | ▯ |

## SAUCES & CONDIMENTS

| | FAT | FIBRE | SUGAR | SALT |
|---|---|---|---|---|
| Brown sauce | | | ▯ | ◊ |
| Piccalilli<br>1oz (28g) | | | | ◊ |
| Sweet pickle<br>1oz (28g) | | | ▯▯ | ◊ ◊ |
| Salad cream<br>1 tablespoon | ◆ ◆ | | | ◊ |
| Tomato purée<br>5oz (142g) tin | | | ▯▯▯ | |
| Tomato ketchup<br>1 tablespoon | | | ▯ | ◊ |

| | FAT | FIBRE | SUGAR | SALT |
|---|---|---|---|---|
| Bovril<br>1 teaspoon | | | | ◊ |
| Curry powder<br>1 tablespoon | ♦ | | | |
| Marmite<br>1 teaspoon | | | | ◊ |
| Oxo cubes<br>1 cube | | | | ◊ ◊ ◊ |

## SOUPS

Manufactured soups contain quite a lot of fat and in the cream soups this will be of the same sort that we found in milk – over half of the saturated kind.

| | FAT | FIBRE | SUGAR | SALT |
|---|---|---|---|---|
| Cream of chicken tinned, 8oz (226g) serving | ♦ ♦ ♦ ♦ | | | ◊ ◊ ◊ ◊ |
| condensed, 8oz (226g) as served | ♦ ♦ ♦ ♦ | | | ◊ ◊ ◊ |
| Chicken noodle dried, as served, 8oz (226g) serving | | | | ◊ ◊ ◊ ◊ |
| Cream of mushroom, tinned, 8oz (226g) serving | ♦ ♦ ♦ ♦ | | | ◊ ◊ ◊ ◊ |
| Minestrone dried, as served, 8oz (226g) serving | ♦ | ✹ | | ◊ ◊ ◊ ◊ |
| Oxtail soup tinned, 8oz (226g) serving | ♦ ♦ | | | ◊ ◊ ◊ ◊ |
| Tomato condensed, as served, 8oz (226g) serving | ♦ ♦ ♦ ♦ | | 🔲🔲🔲 | ◊ ◊ ◊ ◊ |
| cream of, tinned, 8oz (226g) serving | ♦ ♦ ♦ ♦ | | 🔲 | ◊ ◊ ◊ ◊ |

| | FAT | FIBRE | SUGAR | SALT |
|---|---|---|---|---|
| Tomato soup dried, as served, 8oz (226g) serving | ● | | ▦▦ | ◊ ◊ ◊ ◊ |
| Vegetable tinned, 8oz (226g) serving | ● | ✹ | ▦ | ◊ ◊ ◊ ◊ |

## FATS AND OILS

Apart from the low fat spreads, these items are almost 100 per cent fat, and the table on page 52 will show you exactly how much saturated fat they contain.

| | FAT | FIBRE | SUGAR | SALT |
|---|---|---|---|---|
| Butter salted, 10g spread on 1 slice bread | ● ● ● ● | | | ◊ |
| Margarine, all kinds | ● ● ● ● | | | ◊ |
| Low fat spread 10g | ● ● | | | |
| Oils, all kinds, 1 tablespoon | ● ● ● ● ● ● | | | |
| Dripping ½oz (14g) | ● ● ● ● ● ● | | | |
| Lard ½oz (14g) | ● ● ● ● ● ● | | | |
| Suet shredded, ½oz (14g) | ● ● ● ● ● ● | | | |

148

# How the farmers and food industry could help

All the way through this book we've given advice on choosing healthier foods. But there's no doubt that farming policy-makers, food manufacturers, advertisers and food shops could do a great deal more to make the healthier choices the easier choices.

## Starting with fat

- Farming policy could stop creating butter mountains and milk lakes. Over-production of milk puts pressure on the food industry and the public to consume as much as possible.
- Animals bred for meat could be leaner. Instead farmers are encouraged to fatten up lambs, pigs and beef cattle to get higher prices to market.
- Sausage makers could greatly reduce the fat content of their products. Most well-known brands are nearly a quarter fat.
- Similarly, the fat content of most processed meats could be greatly reduced.
- This also applies to ready-made convenience meals.
- A wider range of low fat cheeses would be welcome.
- Food manufacturers could clearly label their products with the fat content (and particularly the *saturated* fat content). They could use a simple symbol system like the one we've devised for Diet 2000. This applies especially to butter, margarine, low fat spreads and cooking fats and oils.

## Turning to sugar

- Food manufacturers could gradually reduce the sugar content of their products and produce a wider range of low sugar alternatives. More tinned fruit could be in natural juice rather than syrup.
- Sugar content could be clearly labelled in terms that everyone can understand.

## Moving on to salt

- Tinned and packet soups, tinned meat products, made-up meals, savoury snacks, bread and cereals, etc, could all be made with much less salt. Manufacturers could make gradual reductions and also introduce more low salt products, as has already happened in the United States and is just beginning in Britain. Cereal manufacturers and bread-makers in particular could try new low salt lines.
- Foods could have their sodium content clearly labelled.

## And finally, fibre

- Bread-makers could increase their range of wholemeal products.
- Breads could be marked with their fibre content.
- Cereal manufacturers could increase their range of wholegrain products.
- More pastry products could be made with wholemeal flour.
- Supermarkets could do more to promote wholefoods.

# Final DIET 2000 reminders

1 Keep an eye on your weight. Don't let it creep up on you!
2 Cut saturated fat in half. Eat less red meat, take the fat off meat; avoid fried and fatty foods; choose lower fat dairy products and spread bread very thinly.
3 Eat more chicken, turkey and fish – all lower in saturated fats.
4 Lose your sweet tooth . . . before you lose them all! Keep sugar to mealtimes only – and then only in moderation.
5 Use salt sparingly. A few crystals can go a long way.
6 Go easy on alcohol. It's lots of liquid calories.
7 Stuff yourself silly with fresh fruit, vegetables, wholemeal bread, potatoes, beans, peas, brown rice, wholemeal pasta and cereal.
8 And now that you care about your health . . . stop smoking.
9 Take plenty of regular exercise.
10 Oh, and have a long and happy life.

# Index to recipes